Beating Childhood Obesity NOW!

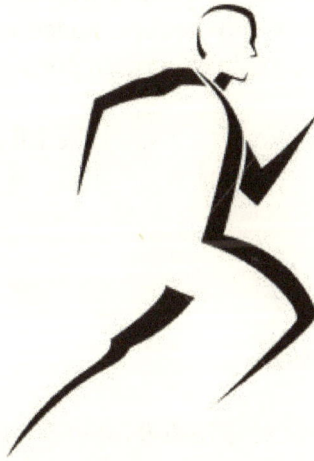

A Simple Solution
for Parents & Educators

Volume I

By Rick Osbourne, MS

Copyright Notices

Dedication

This book is dedicated to the remarkable, resilient, and resourceful renegades who reside (often hiding) within us all. These renegades are strong enough to think for themselves; strong enough to question the status quo; strong enough to challenge the boss, draw their own conclusions, and to live their lives accordingly.

They are not passive products of modern mass production. They refuse to salute the robot. They've successfully repelled indoctrination. And they're less afraid of dying than they are of failing to live while they're still here on planet earth.

In this light I raise a glass to those remarkable, resilient, and resourceful renegades. They have my utmost respect. This world is a better place because of the time they've spent among us.

Table of Contents

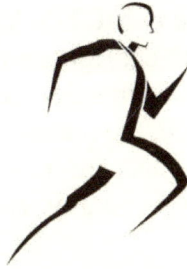

Preface

The 21st century obesity epidemic has proven itself to be the mother load of all epidemics. There's never been another one quite like it before. In that light, one US Surgeon labeled obesity "America's # 1 health threat," and "The terrorist from within." The Pentagon calls it "A national security threat." And the American Association of Actuaries estimates that our nation spends over $270 billion annually on obesity and related problems. With obesity at the root of so many problems, healthcare is destined to bankrupt our nation if we fail to get a handle on this problem pretty soon.

Childhood Obesity

The most insidious aspect of the modern obesity epidemic is what it's doing to our nation's children, to future generations. It undermines everything from their self esteem/confidence, to their social relationships, emotional stability, academic performance, and their school attendance. In the long run it even undermines their future earning potential, their ability to earn a decent living.

As a nation we've been talking about the problem, raising awareness, sharing the vision, and throwing billions of dollars at it without provably moving the needle even slightly for over a decade now. Yet in order to win the obesity war we must get beyond all the talk and begin to ACT PREVENTATIVELY. And in order to act preventatively we must start working with children BEFORE THE OBESITY SEED TAKES ROOT.

Accurately Measuring and Documenting Change

Realistically however, in order to turn the tide on childhood obesity we must first be able to measure body composition changes accurately, and consistently document those changes. And most importantly we must be able to MOTIVATE kids to take stock in themselves, to take action, to eat right and exercise sufficiently in order to avoid the onslaught of this devastating functional disability known as obesity. But to date, the inability to accurately measure, document, and motivate kids has proven to be the Achilles heel of the entire childhood obesity prevention enterprise.

This Book is About...

In this light, the book we've entitled *Beating Childhood Obesity NOW!: A Simple Solution for Parents and Educators* is all about accurately measuring, documenting, and motivating kids to take stock in themselves, and to actively eat and exercise in ways that help make them strong and independent (adult-like) instead of weak and dependent.

Statement of Purpose

This book is a practical, boots on the ground roadmap written for educators who are tired of all the talk, and who are biting at the bit to take preventative action against childhood obesity!

The <u>need is blatantly obvious</u> to anyone who spends any time in public, the local school playground, grocery store, mall, or restaurant, etc. More specifically, one third of Americans are of normal weight, a third are overweight, and another third are obese (per the US Center for Disease Control). The demand for a practical solution is no secret to anyone.

<u>This book will address the problem</u> by showing action oriented educators how easy it can be to help kids arm themselves with the tools they need to fend off America's # 1 health threat – obesity – for life by learning to perform one very simple task, and maintaining the ability for life.

Scope, Organization, and Benefits

Although the concepts we discuss are applicable to kids from 3 to 93, we will limit our focus to kids (as opposed to adults), and we will concentrate most of our time on prevention (where this war is destined to be won) as opposed to rehabilitation (where the war is destined to be lost).

The benefits are so obvious that they hardly need to be pointed out. It prevents millions of kids from being undermined by the modern obesity industrial complex. For educators who are tired of having no practical solution for America's # 1 health threat, this book solves a huge problem. And for the nation's economy it saves billions on the one major item that's driving the national debt right through the ceiling – healthcare.

Unique Features

The most unique feature of this strategy is that, unlike anything else in the market today, IT WORKS! It provides a SYSTEMATIC STRATEGY with which to attack obesity and generate documented evidence starting in the first week of implementation all the way through to completion. At this point participants will have successfully armed themselves against obesity for life by maintaining the ability to physically pull their own weight – which itself demands decent eating and exercise habits. It's simple. It's cheap. And IT WORKS. Now that's pretty unique!

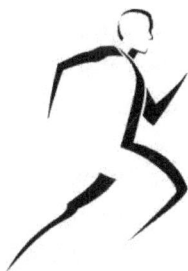

Organization

In the wake of several introductory remarks, this book is organized into seven sections including: The Obstacles to Preventing Childhood Obesity, The Practical Solution, The Supporting Data, The Mechanics, The Motivational Psychology, The Logistics, and The Appendix. The chapters then are organized accordingly within these seven categories.

We lead with the obstacles to success because change is always a challenge. In other words, we're presenting a simple, inexpensive, and viable solution to a problem that for over a decade has been characterized as complicated, expensive, if not overwhelming. The most common reaction is, "It's too simple. It's too good to be true." Conventionalists are heavily invested in the status quo. Getting them to change eyeballs is a hurdle that must be overcome in order to make any real progress.

Section two explores the functional strategy that the American Society of Exercise Physiologists has called "A simple, easily implemented, easily documented, and affordable solution to childhood obesity." It begins with an old coach's observations, follows with a vocabulary designed to speak to kids in ways that they understand. And it ends with an open letter to kids that helps them to recognize that they already know the answer to the problem. So the solution is all about TAKING ACTION.

Section three is designed to answer questions like "Where's your data? Where are your statistics? Where's the empirical, scientific proof that your strategy works?" In reality the answer to these kinds of questions are as plain to see as the nose on your face. They're intuitively obvious to anyone who's ever been on a pull up bar. But for those who argue that reality must be wrapped in numbers, data, and statistics, this section is for you.

Section four is designed to answer questions about the mechanical nuts and the bolts of this simple, functional strategy. What kind of equipment is required? How much does it cost? Where do you start? How do you make progress? Where does nutrition fit into this strategy? How do you know when you've crossed the finish line? This is the only section that includes photos/visuals as part of the explanation so that readers can actually see what it looks like to implement such a project.

Section five is the most important section in the book. Above and beyond anything else this book is about three things. They are motivation, motivation, and motivation. In other words if you can successfully cultivate the motivational flame that exists naturally within all kids and you can keep it alive, you're destined to win. If you fail to cultivate the motivational flame, you're destined to lose. Thus this book is ultimately about motivating and inspiring kids to choose strength over weakness and the principles, when applied correctly, work no matter what the venue.

Section six is dedicated to logistics. How does this strategy fit into my schedule? How much time is required? How do we pay for the tools? Logistics are important and if left unresolved they become an obstacle to success. We want to eliminate the possibility of logistics becoming another excuse for failure. So this section explores, and suggests ways to beat logistical obstacles to success.

Section seven is the Appendix, and it revolves around the pros and cons of a functional alternative to BMI known as a FORE (Functional Obesity Risk Evaluation) Score. The final chapter in the appendix features an endorsement from the American Society of Exercise Physiologists

By the time you finish reading through the Appendix you will have been thoroughly soaked in this simple, functional solution to childhood obesity. And hopefully you'll also be motivated to take action. Otherwise everyone will be wasting their time.

As Gandhi once said "Action exposes priorities." That is to say, talk is only talk. The time has come when we must transform talk into action. That time is now!

Introductory Thoughts on Functional Childhood Obesity Prevention

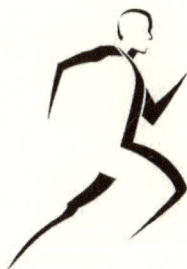

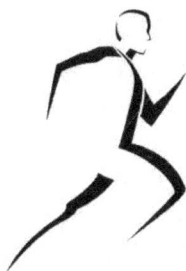

1

Babcock: A Graphic Portrait of the Problem

"Can you remember a spring day in your thirteenth year? A seductive breeze, a few white clouds sketched by a careless artist, the sun striking maddening smells from the moist earth and encouraging unaccustomed pulses in various parts of your body.

It was just such a day in 1972, on a late-morning walk in a small Virginia town that I came across a group of some thirty-five or forty thirteen-year-olds sitting on a grassy bank. I was on a lecture tour, summoned from my motel by the sight and smell of April blossoms.

Standing in front of boys and girls was a taut-muscled young man in gym shoes, gym pants, a white T-shirt, a crew cut, a whistle, and a clipboard. Next to the young man, like a guillotine in the sunlight, was a chinning bar. I stopped to observe the scene.

The man looked at his clipboard. 'Babcock' he called. There was a stir among the boys and girls. One of them rose and made his way to the chinning bar: Babcock the classic fat boy.

Shoulders slumped, he stood beneath the bar. 'I can't,' he said. 'You can try,' the man with the clipboard said.

Babcock reached up with both hands, touched the bar limply –just that-and walked away, his eyes downcast, as all the boys and girls watched, seeming to share in his shame.

I also walked on, flushed with anger. Beneath the anger, I sensed something tentative and hurt. The incident seemed to touch an area of my past that I had conveniently forgotten. The day was so lovely-no time to explore painful areas. I started thinking about other things.

But Babcock was not to let me off so easily. The vignette kept replaying itself in my mind. I was fascinated by the way the fat boy walked to the chin up bar, waddling slightly but moving fast as if eager to have it done with; his condemned stance beneath the bar, the minimal, symbolic touch of his hands on the metal; his utter resignation as he walked away, his head bobbing from side to side.

Again and again, Babcock rose, walked to the bar, stood there, touched the bar, walked off. The scene took on the quality of a Greek drama. The man with the clipboard became the stern-visaged god who devises tests for us, then sends us on without mercy to our respective fates. The boys and girls took the part of the chorus, by their silence condemning the unworthy, and yet by the same silence, expressing their own uneasiness and shame."

...From George Leonard's Classic Book, The Ultimate Athlete

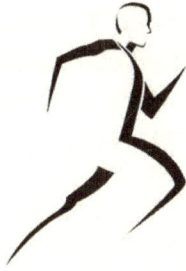

2

My Motivation: An Ode to Teaching

I never feel so strong and confident as when I'm helping kids to find their own strength and confidence. That's my motivation with Operation Pull Your Own Weight.

In a very real sense it's selfish. I'm doing it because I feel so good about myself when I'm doing it. The vibes of appreciation I receive when those kids get stronger and stronger, week after week, and more and more confident in their own natural abilities to set a goal and achieve it in small but relentlessly persistent increments of progress is unique in my life. Under these circumstances, I suddenly feel like Superman, Batman, Spider-man, Indiana Jones, Wyatt Earp, Muhammad Ali, and Elvis all combined in the eyes of these kids. I am unique in their lives.

If I Got This Kind of Lift From...

If I got the same kind of lift from climbing some corporate ladder, from running for public office, or from anything else, I'd be climbing a corporate ladder, running for public office, or doing something else that gives me the same amount of return on my investment of time and effort. But to date, nothing else compares.

There's no thrill of victory like the one I experience when seeing a young boy or girl learning to say "Oh yes I can," in the face of a real challenge, tackling it with unreserved enthusiasm, giving it 110%, having learned, and knowing in their heart of hearts that if they relentlessly persist, they will inevitably cross that finish line.

In the words of the late Winston Churchill, "Never, never, never, never, never, give up!" Not quitting is one very important form of winning. It's not the size of the dog in the fight, but the size of the fight in the dog that counts.

The Moment They Catch Their First Glimpse…

And the moment a child catches their first glimpse of the potential sitting out there on their own personal horizon, as long as they get a little stronger every week, every month, every year, is the moment they start approaching life in a different way, with a different attitude, with an excitement and an enthusiasm that was never there before. Let's just say, "For most everything else there's Master Charge."

And by the way, when I say kids, I'm talking about kids from 3 to 93. The fact of the matter is, when you help someone become stronger and more confident, no matter how old they are, you will have created a relationship that's unique. There aren't that many people in anyone's life who produce that kind of experience. And if you're one of them you will stand out from the crowd. You will hold a unique position in the life of that person, whether they're an elementary school student, or a rock and roll star.

The Clock Keeps on Ticking

So in answer to all those folks who have wondered why the OPYOW clock keeps on ticking inside me, it's because doing it makes me feel so good about me. To repeat my original statement, I never feel so strong and confident as when I'm helping kids to find their own strength and confidence. So there, I've said it out loud. If that were not the case, I'd be unable to persist. The flame would flicker and die. But it has not and now you know why. It's all about me and how it makes me feel about myself.

..

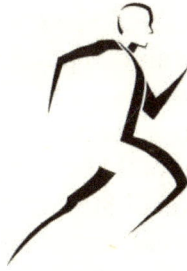

3

The Democratization of Strength in Strongville, IA

Garrison Keillor's legendary boyhood home of Lake Wobegon, MN is the town in which "All the women are strong, all the men are good looking, and all the children are above average." In contrast, Strongville, IA is the town in which all the women are strong, all the men are strong, all the children are strong, and all its citizens strive to grow stronger week after week, month after month, all year long.

More specifically, Strongville is built around the premise that the desire to become stronger (in all kinds of ways) is the natural wellspring of life that must be actively cultivated if its opposites – deterioration, degeneration, and atrophy are to be avoided.

In Strongville it's a matter of honor. It's a moral obligation, a moral imperative to cultivate one's own inborn seeds of strength. It's the source of one's own self-respect as well as one's respect among fellow citizens. Failure to do so is seen as undermining oneself, and in the process undermining one's family, neighborhood, and ultimately the entire town. Thus, what's true for individual citizens is also true for the town itself. Strong, resilient, resourceful, independent citizens are the ingredients that collectively make up a strong, resilient, resourceful, and independent township.*

Life Shaping Habits Start Young

Since all its citizens have physical bodies, Strongville's founding fathers decided that the process of growing stronger should begin with each citizen's physical body. The other thing their founding fathers recognized was the fact that life shaping habits usually begin at a young age. That being the case, they also decided that all Strongville children should be systematically introduced and exposed to the idea of being able to physically pull their own weight (do pull ups) starting in kindergarten.**

They use height adjustable pull up bars in conjunction with a technique called leg assisted pull ups (jumping and pulling at the same time) that together give all Strongville students a place to start, and a way to proceed predictably, in small increments, in front of their friends, towards the end goal of being able to physically pull their own weight.

Naturally Immunized Against Obesity, and...

In over a decade's worth of experience Strongville schools learned that approximately 75% of all students master the ability to physically pull their own weight within one school year. Some take two or even three years. But by the time they walk across the graduation stage, 100% of Strongville High's students are fully capable of physically pulling their own weight.

This means that Strongville High's graduates have naturally immunized themselves against obesity for life as long as they eat and exercise in ways that allow them to maintain the ability to do at least one conventional pull up. You see, as all Strongville citizens know, people who can perform at least one conventional, unassisted pull up can't carry 30% body fat. That is to say, the odds of anyone who can do at least one conventional pull up being obese are remote.

Beyond the Physical

However the physical body is only the beginning of this story. Once students have a solid handle on how to grow physically stronger week after week, month after month, all year long, they apply the same hands-on experiences to subjects like reading, writing, and arithmetic and they grow systematically stronger in these areas as well.

In other words, the experience of growing stronger physically on a regular basis, over time, provides a concrete, tangible foundation upon which to build many new academic skills along with skills in music, art, the political, economic, and social sciences as well.

Seeds of Strength Sewn Far and Wide

When Strongville students finally graduate from high school, head off to college, and eventually pursue employment in various far off places, these walking, talking seeds of strength are sewn and multiplied across the world in places like Chicago, Los Angeles, New York City, Miami, Dallas, New Orleans, Paris, London, Shanghai, and Vienna. Thus the little town and the citizens of Strongville, IA are not only destined to show people around the world how to naturally immunize themselves against obesity for life, but they'll also demonstrate how almost anyone can become strong at everything and weak at nothing by starting with the physical body and building, brick after brick, on a rock solid foundation.

*What's true for townships is equally true for private sector companies/corporations, public sector counties, states, and nations as well.

** The black belt of virtue in Strongville is when one is strong enough to help others cultivate their own respective seeds of strength. In doing so, the individual multiplies and renders infinite his or her own strength building possibilities. In the act of doing so, individuals are effectively experiencing human life on the highest level possible.

22

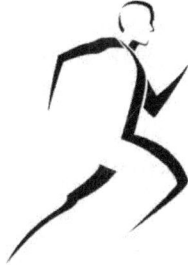

4

I Still Believe in Kids

My staunchly conservative, conventionally patriotic, right leaning friend from suburban Dallas challenged me by saying "So, what do you believe in? You don't believe in the military industrial complex. You don't believe in our education/indoctrination system. You say that big money has corrupted everything from our justice system, to our medical system, our political system, our economic system, and our religious institutions. Exactly who or what do you believe in?"

After quietly sitting through this tea party diatribe I had to take a breath and confess that in my view, it's hard for anyone with both eyes open to believe in much of anything these days. My cynical side was indeed showing through.

The Power of Individual Kids

However, I said there is one thing I still do believe in and that's the power of individual kids – given access to the right information and experiences (which is the fundamental purpose of good parenting and education) – to stand up in the face of daunting challenges, and their innate ability to choose the things they need to do in order to grow stronger, more resilient, more self reliant, despite the cards that are stacked against them every day, every week, every month, and every year of their young lives.

But Most Adults...

On the other hand, I don't feel the same way about most adults. In most cases the indoctrinations have seeped in over time and rooted themselves deeply. The habits are solidly ingrained. They're psychologically, socially, and economically so locked into the system that it's almost impossible for them to see or admit to themselves the degree to which their own lives have been undermined.

And if they can see/admit it, the sheer momentum of the status quo has ground them down and reduced them to the point that they've given up. They've learned to compromise and to accept the tired, old cliché that says, "It's always been this way. You can't fight city hall."

There are of course exceptions to this rule. But they're few and far between. They're the renegades who have refused to swallow the conventional Kool-Aid. But most adults serve as apologists for and guardians of the status quo. They resist change without questioning much of anything. Who has time for questions?

In Answer to My Friend's Question...

So in answer to my friend's question, I still believe in democracy/self governance, social and economic justice, mutual respect (i.e. the golden rule), and enlightened self-interest over greed. And despite the river of toxins we expect them to grow up in today, when given the right information and experiences, I also believe in the power of individual kids to stand up in the face of daunting challenges, and in their innate ability to choose those things that make them strong over those things that make them weak. I've seen it happen too often. That said, I still believe in kids.

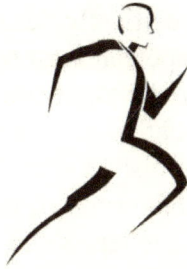

5

The Most Important Lesson Any Kid Can Ever Learn is Best Taught Physically

I contend that one of the most important lessons any kid can ever learn is what I like to call the "Oh yes I can lesson." Whether they're male or female, black, white, yellow, Christian, Muslim, Jew, Asian, European, African, tall, short, rich, poor, or middle class - if kids develop their natural born ability to believe in themselves and to relentlessly persist, odds are they'll learn to succeed, even in the face of life's most difficult challenges, despite a system that's specifically designed to relentlessly mass produce infinite waves of mediocrity, homogeneity, predictability, conventionality, and submission the status quo.

Show 'Em How

Now you may recognize this as the age old American adage that says "You can grow up to be President." But if this lesson is not delivered through practical, hands-on experiences (getting down in the mud and wrestling with the beast), it quickly becomes meaningless, adult doubletalk that goes in one ear and out the other for most kids. In other words talk is cheap. The trick is to show them how to walk the walk if you really expect them to believe in themselves and to live their lives accordingly.

Show 'Em Early

Timing is also an extremely important consideration for the Oh yes I can lesson. In fact you have to get to them before they start school, because conventional school systems are so incredibly efficient at teaching kids the "Oh no you can't lesson."

You see school is specifically designed to pit kids against kids, expecting them to compete against one another for gold stars, teacher's praise, positions in the top reading or math group, who's the prettiest, who's the most athletic, who's the most popular, etc.

By the time they're finished with second grade, most kids will have been thoroughly indoctrinated into the hierarchical mentality that sees the world in terms of a few winners at the top, the bulk of us wrestling around in the middle, and a few stragglers (the kids term these days is losers) bringing up the rear.

Immunizing 'Em Against the Bell Curve

In educational circles it's called the bell curve, and whether it's anywhere near true, most educators are paid to believe it, and to conduct their classes accordingly. If not immunized against this problem before they enter school, kids easily fall pray to the bell curve mentality, and they become passive victims of the machine that's built to convince most kids that they're average or worse, and that there's very little they can do about it.

Conventional educators are of little help because most of them have lived with the bell curve for so long that it's second nature. And once the labels are systematically imbedded it's very difficult for kids to break out of the conventional box and to recognize that the system itself is stacked against them, fatally flawed, if not fraudulent.

However, if you teach kids to think for themselves, to see the world through their own eyes, and to relentlessly persist despite the system, many kids will survive, and their odds of living meaningful lives (real winning) are enhanced a thousand fold. They'll effectively be immunized against the system instead of indoctrinated by it. But remember, one of the biggest keys is to teach kids the Oh yes I can lesson before sending them off to school.

At the Physical Level

The third issue then is how to teach them what you want to teach them. My suggestion is that most young kids are far more physically oriented than they are mentally or spiritually oriented. And it's one thing to tell kids to persist and win, and an entirely different matter to physically show them how to persist and win.

This is true whether they're going to be athletes or first cello in the orchestra. The name of the game in the early years is PHYSICAL!

How About an Example

Ok, how about an example of what I'm talking about here. I suggest that you choose a body weight exercise that's generally associated with being strong. You see all kids want to be strong at everything and weak at nothing. It's in their genes. Have you ever met a kid who wants to be weak at anything? I know I haven't. Once you've chosen the strength oriented body weight exercise, then you simply help your kids learn to master it.

For example, everyone that I know associates pull ups with strength, yet most kids today can't do pull ups. However, if you start them young, before they've had a chance to super-size themselves, most kids can learn to perform pull ups in a very predictable amount (one school year) of time if they get the right advice and have access to the right equipment.

So consider the following scenario. Your patient...
• is going to set a difficult to achieve goal (to perform pull ups)
• is going to be given the right goal achieving information
• is going to be given access to the right goal achieving equipment
• they'll make a little bit of progress every single time they workout
• they'll be congratulated by peers and adults every time they progress (a great motivator!)
• they'll learn to look forward to the opportunity to grab hold of the bar and grow stronger
• within a few months they'll be able to do pull ups (they'll reach their goal)
• they'll be immunized against obesity, because kids who can do pull ups are not obese
• the more pull ups they can do, the leaner they'll be. (Ma Nature designed us that way)
• they'll be physically strong in a way that will impress friends and relatives
• but most importantly they will have learned all the above, first hand, at the physical level
• in other words, they'll have a first hand, physical experience in learning to control (take responsibility for) their own body (the physical self)

Expanding the Oh Yes I Can Lesson

Once this experience has been well chewed, digested, and understood at the physical level it will naturally expand to include everything else in a child's life from their academic work, to their emotional, social (a positive self image is critical), and spiritual possibilities. With patience and relentless persistence, most children can reach almost any goal they set for themselves despite the system that constantly undermines their true potential.

In simplest terms, if you don't think you can, you won't try. And if you don't try, failure becomes a predictable certainty. On the other hand, thinking you can always precedes genuine effort. Once under way, constant progress fans the motivational flames and keeps them burning brightly. And motivation is the fuel that feeds relentless persistence, the key to success.

Soaking it in Yourself

If you physically immunize your kids with the "Oh yes I can lesson," on the physical level before you send them to school, you'll do them the biggest favor possible. You'll teach them the most important lesson they'll ever learn…to persist, persist, and persist again, and again, and again. We call it relentless persistence.

In the words of the late British Prime Minister Winston Churchill, "Never, never, never, never, give up!" In the words of former Olympic mile champion and world record holder Herb Elliot, "You've got to be arrogant enough to think you can, yet humble enough to pay the price."

Reagan, Obama, and the Oh Yes I Can Lesson

On the adult level, former President Ronald Reagan always maintained that his greatest achievement was to make the American people feel better about themselves in the wake of some pretty tough times. Ironically enough we currently have another guy named Obama who's actively preaching the Oh yes we can message to Americans who are again wrestling with some pretty tough times.

And just like their kids, American citizens who are convinced that they're helpless in the face of big money and big government, refuse to invest their limited time and effort into producing change. In other words, they don't try to change things.

And those who fail to try are the conventionalist's best friends. They're easy to control - a dictator's dream.

The Best Time to Start is in Kindergarten

Democracy is completely dependent on citizens who believe that they must govern themselves and control their own lives as opposed to being dictated to by autocratic bureaucrats. In this context, the Oh yes I can lesson lies at the very heart of American Democracy. And the best time to start is in kindergarten.

30

Section 1

Obstacles
to…
Childhood Obesity Prevention Success

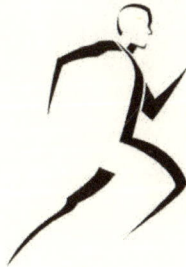

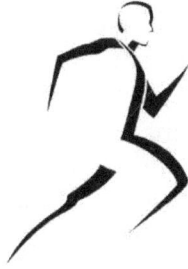

1

Resisting the Modern Obesity Industrial Complex

America's cards are stacked against all kinds of people these days and our kids are no exception to the rule. After listening to medical ethicist Harriet Washington describe what she calls "The medical industrial complex, and reading Dr. Mark Hyman describe "Obesity's toxic triad" (big food, big farming, and big pharma), all of whom are being financially supported by the US Congress (with US tax dollars) in the form of subsidies and loopholes galore, it's easy to conclude that our democratically elected officials in both houses of Congress have been aiding and abetting corporate profiteers at the expense of future generations for some time now.

Why you might ask? Because everyone from the fast food industry to corporate farmers, pharmaceutical companies, colleges, universities, hospitals, and individual doctors are all so financially locked into the system that they can ill afford to rock the boat and tell the American people the truth about anything. And that includes the active role they all play in supporting the root causes of an epidemic the US Surgeon General has called "America's number one health threat," childhood obesity.

Systematic Changes are Unlikely

Presuming the sheer size and momentum of the current system will prevent any significant changes, the question becomes, "What are the odds of systematically arming our kids with the tools they need to stand up and fend off the influences of the obesity industrial complex that's responsible for stacking this deck?

Arming/Activating the Kids Instead

In this light I contend that the odds are excellent – if you know how to do it. Actually the solution is not only simple but it's so inexpensive that individuals from all income levels can afford to partake. On the other hand, done right, it will be extremely expensive to the obesity industrial complex that depends heavily on the epidemic's continuation.

Let me explain by spotlighting one very important fact that most people, if they just think about it for an instant, already know. The fact is, statistics confirm that the odds of an obese person/child being able to do even one conventional pull up are somewhere between miniscule and non-existent.

In other words, if your kids can do at least one pull up, odds are excellent that they're not obese. And furthermore, they'll never have to wrestle with all the problems that follow in obesity's wake – as long as they eat and exercise in ways that allow them to maintain the ability to physically pull their own weight. In short, they will have naturally immunized themselves against obesity for life.

Inspired and Motivated

Furthermore, all kids want to be strong at everything (it's always cool to be strong) and the pull up bar inevitably represents strength to all kids. In this light if you can show kids how to systematically develop the ability to physically pull their own weight and succeed week after week, month after month in front of their friends, you'll be astounded at how motivated most kids become over learning to do pull ups.

Once that goal is achieved it's a simple matter of saying yes to the things that make them strong and no to the things that make them weak. That is to say, on one hand the pull up bar naturally encourages kids choose the fruits and veggies over the pizza and curly fries. On the other hand, it naturally encourages kids to choose active, physical play over sedentary, couch potato inactivity. In other words, it automatically rewards good eating and exercise habits, and automatically punishes poor ones. That's built in.

Undermining the Obesity Industrial Complex

If they test themselves even once a week (10 seconds) in order to make sure their pull up performance remains intact, kids will know for sure that they're winning the war and the obesity industrial complex is losing. In the long run this strategy defunds the culprits, they'll die off for lack of passive victims, and they'll be unable to undermine well armed, pro-activated kids. That's how we can turn the tide and win the war against childhood obesity once and for all. "Action exposes priorities." Gandhi.

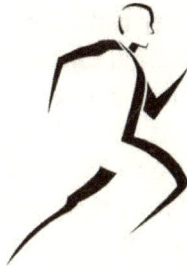

2

The Environmental VS the Functional Approach to Childhood Obesity Prevention

The so called "environmental approach" to resolving childhood obesity is based on the presumption that Johnny, Jimmy, Sally, and Susie are passive reactors to their environment and thus are effectively unable to fend for themselves. Furthermore, if we surround them with an environment overflowing with fast food, sugary drinks, TV, video games, computers, cell phones, Ipods, and no physical education,* then the odds of Johnny, Jimmy, Sally, and Susie falling victim to obesity are increased significantly.

Now I confess, it's hard to argue with these contentions. And to the degree that they're correct the solution automatically becomes changing/improving the environment. So the environmental approach is all about raising awareness ad nauseam (modeled after smoking cessation and seat belt wearing media campaigns), building more public playgrounds in tough neighborhoods, constructing bike paths and sidewalks for residents to use, getting healthy food instead of cheap food into school lunches, eliminating food deserts, forcing fast food chains to stop marketing to kids, and reintroducing physical education into local schools.

Three Big Problems

But the environmental approach is loaded with big problems. The first problem is that it's extremely time consuming to do any, let alone all these things. And in the words of one expert I spoke with recently, "It's going to take a generation to change behavioral patterns." In the meantime millions of American kids are being sucked down the obesity sewer right now while we passively stand around waiting for environmental changes to take place.

The second big problem is that the environmental approach is also extremely expensive. It not only requires decades to implement while undermining millions of kids, but it requires many billions of dollars to pay for the prescriptions suggested by the environmental approach. And all this comes on the heels of a moment in time when many Americans are convinced that our local, state, and national governments are flat broke.

The third problem with this approach is that the solutions prescribed are subject to the whims of those people who have plenty of money, be it corporate philanthropists or government bureaucrats. In other words, the environmental approach by its very nature is a top down, trickle down, propaganda based orientation in which individuals have no real place at the table.

Again, individuals are viewed as passive reactors who (with the exception of taking an occasional market survey) passively react according to predictions if/when the environment changes. All this should be stated along with the fact that such predicted reactions are still little more than speculation. We only hope they'll work.

The Individualistic Trickle Up Approach

In that light let's now have a look at a different approach that's built on a completely different set of presumptions. The individualistic, trickle up, grass roots approach presumes that, given access to the right information and one very simple piece of exercise equipment, most kids not only can, but will systematically transform themselves from passive products of their environments into active agents who help mold and shape the environment in which they live.

Given access to the right opportunities most kids will systematically develop their natural born ability to think for themselves and will actively and naturally choose to do those things that make them strong (like good eating and exercise habits). They'll also actively and naturally choose to avoid those things that make them weak (like bad eating and exercise habits along with tobacco, alcohol, and drug abuse).

Arming Kids Against the System

In other words, given access to the right opportunities most kids will be motivated enough to arm themselves with the tools necessary to fend off the systematic, environmental poisons that they're being asked to grow up with today. Given the right opportunities most kids will develop the physical, mental, emotional, and spiritual strength, the self confidence, the resilience, the resourcefulness, and the dignity required to fulfill their god given potential despite all the environmental challenges they're destined to face.

That is to say, they'll stop waiting around for others to change their world from the top down and they'll do it themselves one kid, one day, one week, and one month at a time. In the process of doing so they'll create the opportunity to develop an entire generation of citizens who are strong enough, bright enough, and resourceful enough to shape their surroundings, their environment in ways that are compatible with Mother Nature and bring a real environmental approach full circle.

*Not to mention drugs, gangs, guns, poverty, and a constant barrage of media violence, sexual innuendo, and bigotry.

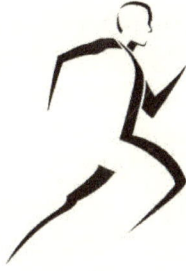

3

A Paradigm Shift From Rehab and Nutrition to Prevention and Functional Performance

Generally speaking, when the topic of childhood obesity comes up, people immediately think of morbidly obese kids. Then the question that automatically pops up is, "What can we do to help those poor kids lose weight?"

In other words, when childhood obesity comes up we automatically think in terms of REHAB, NOT PREVENTION. The tendency is also to presume that those kids who are currently avoiding obesity will continue to avoid it – despite the mountain of evidence predicting the contrary. Why fix something that ain't broke, right?

Furthermore, when the topic of childhood obesity comes up and rehab takes center stage, we have the tendency to think in terms of NUTRITIONAL solutions instead of functional or physical solutions. After all, morbidly obese kids are very limited in what they can do physically because of all the excess weight they carry. That is to say, if they can't run, jump, hop, skip, climb, or play like kids of normal weight, the problem is best approached/initiated from the nutritional perspective.

Conversation Dominated by Rehab and Nutrition

This being the case, when we talk about childhood obesity, rehab and nutrition dominate the conversation at the expense of prevention and function. (1) With these thoughts in mind I suggest that if we expect to turn the tide on this toxic epidemic we must turn the current model on its head, force a paradigm shift, and begin to

41

focus more of our attention on prevention and function, and less of it on rehab and nutrition.

But in All Previous Epidemics...

After all, in previous epidemics including polio, diphtheria, small pox, cholera, and measles, etc., modern science developed vaccines that were designed to strengthen a baby's immune system sufficiently to fend off the causes of these dread diseases. If we'd failed to do this we'd still be wrestling with epidemics in polio, diphtheria, etc. That is to say, modern scientists triumphed over these epidemics precisely BECAUSE they focused their attention PRIMARILY on PREVENTION.

The Question Becomes...

In this light the question becomes, "What can we do for kids, starting at a young age in order to arm them with the tools they need to actively fend off obesity, and all the problems that follow in its wake - for a lifetime? What can we do to PREVENT obesity in ways that are similar to the ways we've prevented polio, diphtheria, small pox, etc.? More specifically, to the degree that we PREVENT obesity, we systematically REDUCE the need to deal with rehab - just like with polio, diphtheria, and small pox.

Now let's recognize that in a very fundamental sense, obesity is itself a functional disability, no different from a torn ACL or a rotator cuff injury. There are many things that obese kids are unable to do BECAUSE of their excess weight. Examples we sited earlier include running, jumping, hopping, skipping, and climbing a rope or a tree.

One other thing obese kids can't do is conventional pull ups. More scientifically stated, the odds of obese kids being able to do even one pull up are about the same as winning the lottery or getting hit by lightening. The logical flip side of this statement is that the odds of KIDS WHO CAN DO conventional pull ups being obese are also about the same as winning the lottery or being hit by lightening.

One Really Simple Solution

Therefore, one simple (cost effective/cheap) way to prevent obesity is to begin young (K-5 where obesity levels are predictably lower) and help kids learn to physically pull their own weight. Once

they've accomplished this goal make sure they know that if they eat
and exercise in ways that allow them to maintain the ability to do
pull ups, odds are they will NEVER experience America's # 1
health problem, obesity, or the problems (type 2 diabetes, heart
problems, social and economic issues, etc.) that are rooted in it.

1. This is not to say that prevention and exercise are totally ignored.
They're not. But they are relegated to the back of the bus in favor of
rehab and nutrition which is a major league, strategic mistake that
undermines future generations.

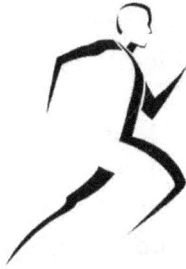

4

Reframing Childhood Obesity in Order to Win

When framing an issue you're basically deciding what's more important (that goes inside the frame and gets the attention) and what's less important (that goes outside the frame and is effectively ignored). Done right, framing prioritizes information. It gives an issue context, meaning, and clarification.

When it comes to the issue of childhood obesity prevention framing the issue correctly is absolutely essential if we're ever to understand it, be able to accurately measure changes, eventually turn the tide and win the war on this 21st century plague. Let's check out the three framing possibilities currently being used today.

Frame # 1

If you're an exercise physiologist you've been taught to frame the issue of obesity in terms of a concept known as body composition and to express it according to another concept known as percentage of body fat. You've also been taught that obesity is defined as anyone whose percentage of body fat is 30 or above. Between 25 and 30 is defined as overweight. Between 20 and 25 is defined as normal. And under 20 is defined as underweight. Furthermore all this is accurate and scientifically sound.

Frame # 2

On the other hand, if you're a public health official or an actuary who crunches numbers on behalf of a health insurance company you've been taught to frame obesity in terms of massed averages and to express obesity according to a concept known as Body Mass Index – BMI for short. The formula for BMI (body weight/height squared X 703) however asks nothing about an individual's body fat or muscle mass – the only two ingredients that count for the exercise physiologist's body composition concept.

Conflict Between Frames # 1 and # 2

Thus there's an inherent conflict between these two conventional orientations to obesity measurement. In this light public health officials (including the CDC) are often quick to admit that BMI was originally intended to assess large populations, so it's probably inaccurate for assessing an individual's level of obesity. But then what's a group if not a collection of individuals? There's also a motivational void with both orientations since to most kids, BMI and Percentage of Body Fat are abstract and meaningless.

Frame # 3

Finally, if you're a physical therapist you've been taught to frame your issues in terms of improving your clients' functional performance. If an athlete comes to you in the wake of arthroscopic knee surgery, for example, your job is to help that player re-gain the functional potential of their injured knee so they can walk, run, jump, and play again. In other words, the question for the PT is "What can you do right now? That's the baseline. And then, "What can we do in order to gradually improve the stabilization, the functional quality, and thus the performance of the injured knee?"

Direct Relationship Between Body Fat and Performance

So when it comes to childhood obesity PT's focus on functional change instead of BMI or Percentage of Body Fat. If a kid is running faster and further, if they're jumping higher, if they're moving more quickly from side to side on the playground, if they're climbing higher on the rope, doing more pull ups, bar dips, etc, you have cold, hard, empirical evidence that these kids are making progress in terms of body composition. They're losing fat, gaining muscle, or both. After all, if it was not for this very direct relationship between physical performance and percentage of body fat, nobody would give a hoot about body composition at all.

It's All About Motivation

But the most important benefit of framing obesity in terms of functional performance is that kids understand it in a way they don't understand BMI or PBF. And when they experience regular and tangible payoffs in functional terms, they're also motivated to eat better and exercise more in order to keep on keeping on.

Getting stronger in front of your friends is cool. Kids love it. And their motivational flames burn hotter under these conditions. And when it comes to obesity prevention, the bottom line in our view is all about motivation. If we can light that motivational flame and help it grow, everyone wins. If we fail to light the motivational flame and it dies out, everyone loses. It's about that simple.

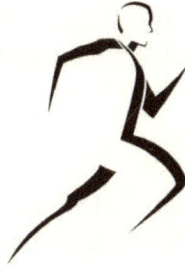

5

The Challenge of Validating BMI

The concept of body mass index (BMI for short) is omnipresent in the field of childhood obesity these days. It seems to be so universally accepted by the medical community, academia, and the insurance industry, etc. that you seldom, if ever hear anyone question its validity. And it's the metric upon which an entire epidemic has been built.

So in this commentary we'd like to play the devil's advocate and pose the question, how can we scientifically confirm (or refute) the validity of BMI? Since BMI is suppose to be a reflection of body composition (body fat VS muscle mass), validation would logically require that BMI be compared to any one of the other three conventionally accepted body composition testing methods in order to see to what degree it yields the same or at least similar feedback.

The Skin Fold Method

For example you could compare BMI readings to the skin fold method of testing body composition. This method requires a knowledgeable technician to use a skin fold caliper designed to measure the skin thickness at various points on a subject's body. The data gathered is placed into a formula which in turn spits out a percentage of body fat. If that number is 30 or higher, the subject is labeled obese. If it's between 25 and 30 they're overweight. If it's below 25 they're considered normal.

One problem with this strategy is that it is labor intensive, time consuming, and expensive enough that it's almost cost prohibitive to use in schools. The other (even bigger) problem is that you can have 5 different technicians testing the same person and often you'll get 5 different readings. In other words, if the validity of the skin fold method itself is itself questionable, basing the validity of BMI on its ability to match another problematic technique lends little to its validity.

Bio Electronic Impedance

So what if you compared BMI to another conventionally accepted method of body comp measurement known as bio-electronic impedance? Bio-electronic impedance is the computerized entry in the body comp measurement derby that fires electronic current through the body in order to reflect a subject's percentage of body fat.

The problem with this strategy is that electronic impedance has a hard time distinguishing between fat and water. So if you're one of those well hydrated people who are constantly drinking bottled water during the day, (or chronically dehydrated) the odds of getting an accurate reading are not good. Furthermore, if the validation of electronic impedance happens to be based on comparisons to the skin fold method or BMI you automatically create an inbreeding issue because of their inherent flaws.

Underwater Weighing

But what if you compared BMI to the results of underwater weighing, the gold standard technique most favored by exercise physiologists in the lab? Underwater weighing compares your body weight on land to your body weight under water. Since fat weighs less than water it's buoyant. The difference between the two figures is fat. So for example, if you weight 160 lbs on land and 120 lbs under water, you're carrying 40 lbs of fat. Dividing 40 by 160 reveals that 25% of your body is made up of fat.

The problem with this strategy is that the time and expense (it's significantly more expensive than either bio-electonic impedance, or the skin fold method) required to get it done dictates that this comparison has most likely never occurred. The second problem is that if the subjects being tested fail to blow all the air out of their lungs when they're under water (a challenging task for most humans) the underwater weighing test is invalidated because air weighs less than water too and it's mistakenly construed as fat.

Validity Problems Galore

As it turns out, validity problems are rampant when it comes to testing body composition. In order to validate any one method based on another problematic method makes no logical sense. The question at this point becomes, is there any way to measure body composition accurately and cost effectively so that we know with any degree of confidence that Johnny, Jimmy, Sally, or Susie are winning, losing, or spinning their wheels when it comes to the war on childhood obesity?

By Reverse Engineering...

The answer as it turns out is yes...if you're willing to back into the problem and ask "What's the purpose of body composition testing in the first place?" Why would anyone care if their percentage of body fat was 20, 25, 30, or 35? By themselves these are only numbers floating around in a meaningless void.

In that light, the main reason that anyone would prefer to have a 20% body fat reading over a 30% body fat reading is that FAT IMPAIRS FUNCTION. If an athlete gains 10 pounds of fat their ability to run, jump, move quickly from side to side will automatically be reduced. If a senior citizen gains 10 pounds of fat their ability to get up and down a flight of stairs or in and out of an easy chair is also automatically reduced. On the other hand, if the athlete or a senior citizen loses 10 pounds of fat their functional performance automatically improves.

That's why changes in body composition matter. That's why they're important. If changes in body composition did not automatically reflect changes in functional performance nobody would care anything about body composition.

Validating or Invalidating BMI

Now, with all this in hand let's revisit the original question regarding the validity of BMI. If we agree that body composition changes automatically reflect functional performance changes we can test and see if improved BMI readings reflect improved abilities to run, jump, climb a rope, get up and down a flight of stairs or out of an easy chair, etc. To the degree that BMI changes accurately reflect functional performance changes, BMI can legitimately be validated or invalidated.

For that matter we can and should do the same with the skin fold, electronic impedance, and underwater weighing techniques. Doing so would tell us how valid or invalid these conventional methods are as well.

Systematically Undermining Progress
In the meantime it's the contention of this essay that our inability to accurately measure changes in body composition systematically undermines our ability to make legitimate progress in the war against childhood obesity. That is to say, if we're unable to accurately measure changes in body composition we'll continue to have no idea if an intervention is winning, losing, or falling somewhere in between.

Furthermore, we contend that all body composition measurement tools can and should be validated or invalidated by comparing their feedback to changes in functional performance. Until we can legitimately measure changes in obesity levels we'll continue wrestling unsuccessfully with childhood obesity and paying the price for failing to understand what we're doing.

Let's Try Asking the Right Questions...
Now, since the primary virtue of any body composition reading is found in its ability to predict functional performance (for better or worse), the following are representative of the kinds of questions that need to be asked and answered.

1. Does an improved/lower percentage of body fat score via BMI accurately predict one's ability to run faster, jump higher, or function more efficiently?**

2. Does an improved/lower percentage of body fat score via skin fold accurately predict an improved ability to perform pull ups, bar dips, or hand stand push ups?

3. Does a low percentage of body fat score via electronic impedance accurately predict a high capacity for learning pull ups, bar dips, and rope climbing?

4. Does a high percentage of body fat score via under water weighing accurately predict a low capacity for learning pull ups, bar dips, and rock climbing?

5. Does an improved ability to run, jump, climb a rope, do pull ups, bar dips, or hand stand push ups accurately predict an improved BMI, skin fold, bio-electronic impedance, or under water weighing score?

6. And if they do not, then why would anyone care anything about any one of these four conventional methods of body composition measurement?

7. Most importantly, are kids inspired and motivated by abstract body composition readings of any kind? Or are they inspired and motivated by performance gain?

*BMI is the metric of choice not because of its accuracy, but because on the front end it's so much cheaper than any of the other three conventional testing methods. But BMI's role in undermining progress has made it extremely expensive in the long run.

** Instead of running and jumping, the appropriate test for older folks might be getting up and down a flight of stairs, or in and out of an easy chair.

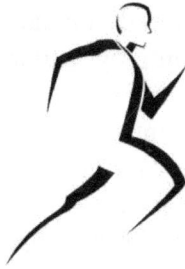

6

Show Me Your Data: 3 Simple Scenarios

As an active and outspoken proponent of testing body composition changes according to changes in functional performance, I've often heard the challenge, "Show me the data. Show me the statistics. Show me the empirical evidence, the proof" from various guardians of the status quo.

Mind you this challenge inevitably comes from people who've never questioned the validity of BMI. After all, BMI is universally accepted in the conventional medical community, so why question it...right?

In answer to those challenges I offer the following data, stats, proof. Check them out and you'll see why you might want to question the validity of BMI.

Scenario # 1:
• Person A GAINS 10 lbs of body fat and their BMI deteriorates.
• Person B LOSES 10 lbs of body fat and their BMI improves
• Person C GAINS 10 lbs of muscle mass and their BMI DETERIORATES
• Person D LOSES 10 lbs of muscle mass and their BMI IMPROVES
• Person E works hard and REPLACES 10 lbs of body fat with 10 lbs of muscle mass and their BMI REMAINS CONSTANT...NO CHANGES AT ALL

Scenario # 2:
• Person A GAINS 10 lbs of body fat and their pull up performance (along with their running, jumping, and ability to move quickly) automatically deteriorates.

• Person B LOSES 10 lbs of body fat and their pull up performance (along with their running, jumping, and ability to move quickly) automatically improves.
• Person C GAINS 10 lbs of muscle mass and their pull up performance (along with their running, jumping, and ability to move quickly) automatically improves.
• Person D LOSES 10 lbs of muscle mass and their pull up performance automatically deteriorates.
• Person E works hard and REPLACES 10 lbs of body fat with 10 lbs of muscle mass and their pull up performance improves dramatically.

Two Questions for the Status Quo Guardians
In this light my first question to the guardians of the status quo becomes, have YOU personally ever seen the data that validates BMI? The answer is inevitably no, because THEY (whoever they are?) have done all the research. And who are WE to question the validity of the data that THEY universally support. The emperor's new clothes are spectacular indeed, are they not?
My second question is, given the choice between scenario # 1 and scenario # 2 which one makes the most sense to you? Anyone who's seriously considered the concept of BMI is well aware of the dilemma posed by scenario # 1 and scenario # 2 and the answer to the second question becomes a "no brainer."

Scenario # 3:
With all this info in hand I'd now like to offer a third set of statistics for those who'd like to taste the data, the proof, the empirical evidence for a functional alternative.
• 492 elementary school age students
• 290 boys and 202 girls
• The only qualifier was that all members of this group were able to do at least one conventional pull up/chin up.
• BMI's were run on the entire group of 492 students.
• Of the 202 girls 0% had BMI's of 30 or above. Most were in the lower 20's.
• Of the 290 boys, 98% had BMI's of 30 or above. Most were in the lower 20's.

56

• Of the 2% of boys who had BMI's of 30 or above NONE were hydrostatically weighed in the wake of the testing.
• I speculate if this had been done the hydrostatic weighing would have identified these students as the "linebackers" in the group. They would have been bigger boned and heavier muscled and their body comps would have been less than 30%, which is to say they were not really obese – despite their BMI scores.

The Bottom Line

The bottom line in my view is that any body comp measurement that's worthy of serious consideration must automatically and accurately predict/reflect changes in functional performance. If it fails to do this the measurement is little more than a mathematical abstraction floating around in space without value or meaning to anyone. That being the case the question becomes, why not go directly to functional performance change in order to get an accurate reflection of changes in body composition?

With all that said, I personally support a concept called BMI + FORE (an acronym for Functional Obesity Risk Evaluation).

58

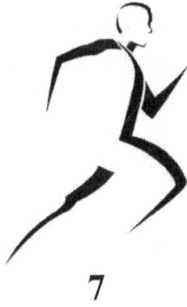

7

Your Strategy Has No Aerobic Component

Like all new ideas, Operation Pull Your Own Weight has encountered its share of criticisms. One of the most frequent is, "But Coach, your program has no aerobic component. You're not getting anyone's heart rate up into the target heart rate zone and keeping it there for 15 or 20 minutes like the Cooper Clinic has preached about for the better part of 40 years. That means you have an incomplete fitness program."

The Critics are Right, But...

My initial reaction is to say you're right. Despite the fact that we encourage active lifestyles that burn calories and keep kids light, OPYOW is an incomplete fitness program. On the other hand, we've never implied anything else. It's nothing more (and nothing less) than a functional acid test that guarantees those who can perform pull ups that they're naturally immunized against obesity for life as long as they maintain the ability.

In other words the critics are absolutely right to say that, by virtue of having no aerobic component, OPYOW does almost nothing to directly strengthen the heart. And the heart is a pretty important organ for most of us. They are also right to say that pull ups burn very few calories. I mean, I agree with anyone who claims that a walk around the block burns more calories than pull ups.

They're Also Wrong

On the other hand they're dead wrong to imply that OPYOW is not heart friendly. You see to the degree that this strategy minimizes excess weight, it also decreases the workload on the heart 24 hours a day 7 days and week...and that's no small consideration.

59

Let me say it another way. I can show you plenty of obese kids who can walk around the block. I can also show you plenty of obese kids who can get their heart rates up into the target zone and keep 'em there for enough time to directly strengthen their hearts.

Imagine That

However, odds are that nobody can show me (or anyone else) even one obese kid (one obese human being) who can perform pull ups. You see those two qualities are mutually exclusive and they almost never occupy the same physiological territory. Where you find one you will not find the other. OPYOW is a functional acid test that immunizes kids against obesity for life. That being the case, a more heart friendly program would be hard to imagine. Imagine that.

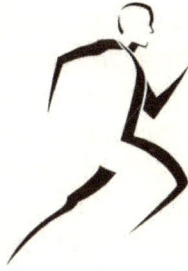

8

Profiting From Childhood Obesity Prevention?

When it comes to getting things done, everything boils down to priorities. When (or if) an item gets to the top of the stack it gets your attention and the odds of getting it done improve dramatically. On the other hand, if an item never gets to the top of the stack the odds of getting it done are effectively nonexistent.

Now when it comes to priorities they come in two distinct varieties. There are priorities that generate profit, and there are priorities that generate no profit. And for most people who live and work in the real world of economic necessity, the odds of taking action on profit generating priorities are significantly higher than the odds of taking action on priorities that generate no profit. ("Action exposes priorities" Gandhi.)

Almost Nobody Gets Paid for Childhood Obesity Prevention

With that said, welcome to the world of childhood obesity. We're talking about the epidemic the US Surgeon General has labeled "America's number one health threat." We're also talking about an epidemic that almost nobody gets paid to prevent. There's lots of talk, lots of awareness raising, vision sharing, health fairs, four color flyers, TV spots, and even events held on the White House lawn.

But to find actual boots on the street, to find real live adults working with real live kids on preventing obesity – well suffice it to say that you should avoid holding your breath while trying to find one. I'm not saying they don't exist. They do exist. But they're few and far between and thus extremely hard to find.

Pediatricians and Teachers

Think about it. Pediatricians get paid for preventing polio, small pox, diphtheria, whooping cough, and measles so those things all get done on a systematic basis. But pediatricians don't get paid to prevent the epidemic that dwarfs all these previous epidemics combined – childhood obesity – so they don't get that done.

Teachers get paid to teach math, science, English, social studies, chemistry, biology, physics, and even physical education, so they get all those jobs done. But teachers don't get paid to prevent childhood obesity, so they don't get that job done.

YMCA's, Boys and Girl's Clubs, Scouts...

YMCA's, Boys and Girls Clubs, Boy Scouts, Girls Scouts, and park districts all hire people (or recruit volunteers) to occupy/entertain kids after school and during the summer while moms and dads hold down jobs that enable them to pay the bills. But with rare exceptions, these organizations don't hire people and charge them specifically with the task of preventing childhood obesity. So despite all the lip service these organizations pay to childhood obesity prevention, it fails to get done in these organizations as well.

If There Was a Profit Generated...

I once heard the great Bill Russell (of Boston Celtics fame) address an auditorium full of college students at Northern Illinois University on the topic of race relations back in the late 60's. He started out by observing "If there was a profit to be generated in resolving the issue of race relations, it would be resolved tomorrow." Unfortunately childhood obesity occupies exactly the same boat today. In fact in the latter's instance the financial incentives are stacked against finding a solution because the obesity industrial complex is making so much money on the problems of obese people.

Getting Paid for Generating Real Value

Thus the moral of this story is, when professionals, including physical educators, family doctors, chiropractors, osteopaths, pediatricians, nurses, etc. find ways to generate profits from preventing childhood obesity, it will become a priority that demands our attention and that actually gets done. But until that transformation occurs, childhood obesity will remain one of those "extremely important priorities" to which we pay lip service, but we never really get around to doing anything about.

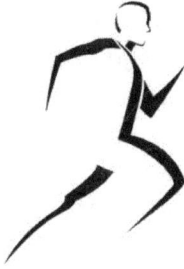

9

Paying to Prevent America's # 1 Health Threat?

Here's a novel idea. How about we start paying people to prevent childhood obesity? After all, there's an army of doctors/nurses in every state who are being paid to vaccinate and immunize kids against polio, small pox, diphtheria, cholera, and measles. That is to say doctors are being paid to PREVENT these diseases from happening, and over time our nation has effectively eliminated these epidemics from our shores.

In contrast the raging childhood obesity epidemic that's been labeled America's # 1 health threat by the US Surgeon General, a national security threat by the Pentagon, and an annual $270 billion dollar drain on the economy by the Society of Actuaries, has no comparable army working to prevent it. To find anyone anywhere who's being paid to PREVENT childhood obesity is like hunting for the proverbial needle in the haystack.

Yah But...

That's not to say the public health sector lacks employees whose titles include the terminology "childhood obesity prevention." Those people exist, but their main functions are to "raise awareness, pass out literature at local Chamber of Commerce meetings, or conduct BMI screenings at local health fairs, etc.

But ironically, nobody is being paid to get down into the trenches and prevent obesity in the way that doctors/nurses are being paid to prevent polio, small pox, diphtheria, cholera, and measles. In the real world you only get what you pay for.

So, Why is This the Case?

So, why are we in this dilemma? Currently there are no pills, shots, or vaccines that strengthen the human immune system in such a way that we fend off obesity like we fend off polio, diphtheria, and small pox. In other words, without a vaccine medical practitioners are at a loss when it comes to systematically arming kids with the tools they need to fend off obesity. As the result, nobody actually gets paid to prevent obesity.

One Simple Observation

With these thoughts in mind, I offer the following observation. It's common knowledge that, due to their excess weight, obese kids are unable to do lots of things that normal weight kids can do. And one of those things obese kids can't do is conventional pull ups. The logical flip side of this observation is that the odds of kids who CAN do pull ups being obese are about the same as winning the lottery.*

In Families for Example

So what can we conclude from this simple observation? We can conclude that the odds of kids who can physically pull their own weight of being obese are negligible. If parents want their kids to be functionally immunized against obesity (and all the problems that follow in its wake) help them learn to do pull ups. Then urge them to eat and exercise in ways that allow them to maintain the ability forever. But leaving obesity prevention in the hands of parents is not a systematic solution to the problem.

In Schools for Example

In the school setting we can conclude that the more kids we have who are able to physically pull their own weight, the fewer kids we'll have with obesity problems. Is there a school in the entire US who can't afford to help students learn to do this? And if we actually paid Physical Educators (for example) to accept this challenge, we'd eliminate obesity from our schools in less than a decade. This scenario thus qualifies as a SYSTEMATIC SOLUTION to the problem.

But Only If...

This same strategy could be carried out in any number of venues. It could happen in the local YMCA, Boys and Girls Clubs, Scouts, churches, not to mention in the offices of pediatricians, physical therapists, and chiropractors just to name a few. But if we're in the market for a SYSTEMATIC SOLUTION, don't expect it to happen until people are actually being paid to address the problem. Everything else is just more talk.

*The same thing can be said for rope climbing, bar dips, hand stand push ups, single legged squats among others. In some circles these are known as functional acid tests that if mastered, reduce the odds of obesity dramatically.

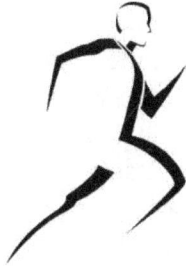

10

The Role Empirical Science Plays in Preventing Childhood Obesity

I contend that my nose is located on my face. There have never been any scientific studies or statistics wrapped around this intuitively obvious fact. But my 65 years of life experience has led me to that conclusion and I've never been inclined to question it. And until someone makes it their business to prove me wrong I will continue to accept this as an empirically provable (i.e. accessible to the senses) fact that requires no debate.

Pull Ups VS Obesity

In a similar sense, and speaking as a former Physical Educator/coach (17 years worth) I've never seen an obese kid (30% body fat or more) who could perform even one conventional, unassisted pull up. On the other hand, any kid who could perform at least one pull up was inevitably, relatively strong and light.

In other words, for all practical purposes they were never obese. Furthermore, I've discussed this matter with thousands of colleagues as well as lay people and none of them has ever seen or heard of an obese kid who could do pull ups.

One possibility (the ability to do a pull up) simply excludes the other (obesity). My 65 years of life experience has also led me to that conclusion. And like the nose on my face, until someone makes it their business to prove the intuitively obvious wrong, I will continue to accept this as an empirically provable fact that requires no debate.

The Earth was Flat Argument

But then my friends in the "scientific community" are quick to point out that there was a time when the Earth being flat was conventionally accepted as a fact. That was before scientists came along in order to set the record straight. In other words, the intuitively obvious is not always true...right?

On this point I can't disagree with my scientific friends. The intuitively obvious is not always true and that's been proven over and over again by science. On the other hand, whether discussing the nose on my face or the earth being flat, the intuitively obvious has always been given the benefit of the doubt, and has been accepted as empirical fact until some scientist comes along and proves it to be otherwise.

The Burden of Proof is on Them, Not...

With all that said, I'm perfectly open to the possibility that my intuition could be dead wrong when it comes to the relationship between pull ups and obesity. But unless I misunderstand the scientific method, the burden of proof falls on those who contend otherwise, and not on those of us whose life experiences collectively support the intuitively obvious experience that says the ability to perform at least one pull up excludes the possibility of the performer carrying 30% body fat/being obese.

Until that burden of proof is met, I'll continue to contend (along with all my friends) that the odds of an obese kid being able to do even one unassisted pull up are somewhere between microscopically small and non-existent (and vice versa). Furthermore, I'll contend that this claim is a scientific fact, every bit as obvious and provable as my nose being on my face.

I Hereby Challenge Science...

In conclusion, I'd like to take this opportunity to CHALLENGE the scientific community including the US Center for Disease Control, the American Medical Association, the American College of Sports Medicine, the American Association of Pediatrics, the Food and Drug Administration, along with scientists and experts from higher institutions of learning such as Harvard, Yale, Stanford, and the University of Chicago, Dr. Oz, Dr. Sanjay Gupta, Jamie Oliver, and ANONE ELSE who's legitimately interested in resolving the childhood obesity epidemic that's costing so many kids so much, to DISPROVE this intuitively obvious relationship. And while you're at it, PROVE that BMI means anything to anybody when it comes to body composition change…the one thing that must improve if we're to turn the tide on obesity.

P.S. For those in the scientific community who claim to be data driven and who insist on statistics before you buy into the intuitively obvious, we have a 492 subject study which overwhelmingly confirms the claim that the odds of kids who can do at least one pull up being obese are microscopically small. If you're legitimately interested, check out the following.

• According to The US Center for Disease Control (US CDC), 17% (or 12.5 million) of all US kids between the ages of two and nineteen are obese.

• Compare the US CDC data to the following 492 kid study containing BMI data from 290 boys and 202 girls (2nd, 3rd, and 4th graders) who's ONLY qualification was, THEY COULD ALL DO AT LEAST ONE UNASSISTED PULL UP.

• According to this 492 kid study/bar graph, 0% (i.e. NONE) of the 202 GIRLS were obese, which is another way of saying, 100% WERE NOT OBESE!

• According to this same 492 kid study/bar graph, 2% of the 290 BOYS were obese while 98% WERE NOT OBESE.

• Therefore this empirical data overwhelmingly supports the intuitively obvious claim that says the odds of kids who can perform at least one conventional pull up being obese are somewhere between microscopically small and non-existent.

• Now imagine what happens to the odds of them ever becoming obese if we helped those 37,500,000 (50,000,000 minus 12,500,000) kids who are not obese learn to do at least one unassisted pull up and encouraged them to maintain it. Can you say PREVENTION?

• Then imagine what happens if we help those 12,500,000 kids who are obese learn to perform at least one unassisted pull up. Can you say ELIMINATION?

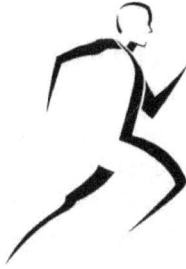

11

Moving the Mountains of Conventionality

It's a mountain and it sneers at the mere thought of ever being moved. It's conventional, traditional, the window through which almost everyone views the problem. The medical establishment has bought in. The education establishment has bought in. The insurance industry has bought in. Municipal, county, and state governments have bought in. And the federal government and its myriad of agencies have all bought in.

Is it even possible that they're all wrong? And if they recognized it, is it possible that they'd have the courage to fess up and admit the error of their ways? After all, we're talking about "the experts" here. They all have degrees from respected institutions of higher learning. And it's humiliating for experts to say anything like, "I guess I missed that one. I blew it. I've been wrong all these years because I followed the herd instead of thinking for myself. I'm an accomplice." Is it possible that the emperor is standing smack dab in the middle of town square wearing no clothes?

The BMI Mountain

The emperor or the mountain we're talking about in this case is the concept upon which the entire childhood obesity epidemic has been built – BMI. It's omnipresent and everywhere when it comes to measuring changes in obesity. The AMA endorses it. The ACSM endorses it. The CDC and the AAP endorse it. The Republicans, the Democrats, and the Libertarians endorse it. They've all laid their own political capital, their hard won reputations on the line on behalf of BMI.

73

Despite the Indisputable Fact That...

This is the case despite the indisputable fact that if I work out real hard for a period of time and gained 10 lbs of sheer muscle mass, my functional performance, physical efficiency, body composition, and metabolism all improve dramatically, while my BMI deteriorates significantly. If I got lazy and lost 10 lbs of muscle mass, my functional performance, physical efficiency, body composition, and metabolism all deteriorate significantly while my BMI improves.

On the other hand, if I replace 10 lbs of fat with 10 lbs of muscle, my BMI remains exactly the same. If I replace 10 lbs of muscle with 10 lbs of fat, my BMI is completely static. There's absolutely no difference in either case.

Nothing, Nada, Zilch...

In other words, BMI tells you absolutely nothing about changes in muscle mass or body fat – the ONLY two things that count when addressing the issue of obesity. Yet when pressed with this kind of evidence, this cold, hard, empirical data, very few members of the conventional establishment have the courage, let alone the candor to admit that the emperor is wearing no clothes.

After all, they're being paid by the emperor to agree with the emperor. They're being paid to be the guardians of the status quo. Their credibility is at stake. This mountain has no intention of moving anywhere.

The Audacity to Challenge

So when anyone has the audacity to challenge the credibility of the mountain, and offers a viable alternative, that person is never welcomed with open arms. In fact that person is initially ignored, told to go away, to mind his own business. If/when that fails, the experts say he lacks the scientific evidence to challenge the mountain/the emperor.

When the challenger points out that BMI undermines all childhood obesity prevention interventions that are BMI based, the experts squeeze their eyes tightly shut. When he points out that BMI undermines the life quality of 10 million American kids the experts place their hands over their ears. When he points out the inability to resolve the obesity epidemic costs America $270 billion annually, the experts stand up and quickly walk away.

It's blasphemous. It's anathema. And it threatens the virtue and stability of the status quo – not to mention its profitability. It's insightful to recognize that, in the end everything boils down to the quarterly profits. Astonishing!

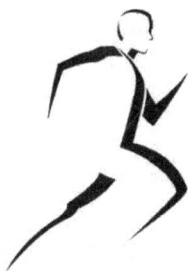

12

The Old Hag VS the Beautiful Young Woman

It's all packed into one picture/drawing, the ugly old hag, and the beautiful, young woman. Both are present in the same drawing, one effectively hiding in plain sight. But if you focus on the old hag, you'll be unable to simultaneously see the beautiful young woman. Conversely, if you focus on the beautiful young woman, you'll be unable to simultaneously see the old hag.

Psychologists suggest that what you're able to see is heavily dependent on what you expect to see. Thus if you expect to see the old hag, then the old hag is what you'll see. On the other hand, if you expect to see the beautiful young woman, the beautiful young woman is what you'll see.

How Does That Apply to OPYOW?

Now, what in the world does this well known optical illusion have to do with Operation Pull Your Own Weight? As it turns out, a lot! If you're thoroughly soaked in and effectively indoctrinated by the omnipresent suggestion that childhood obesity is an extremely complicated problem with multiple causes, then it stands to reason that it requires extremely complicated, sophisticated (and so expensive) solutions. That's what you'll expect to hear when someone talks about solutions to this problem.

Under these presumptions, when someone offers a solution that's simple, functional, naturalistic, and affordable, it's almost impossible to see because it contradicts your expectations. If, upon hearing the term childhood obesity you automatically slip into a weight watcher's mode and you view the problem from a rehab perspective, then it's almost impossible to see a solution that's built on prevention. If you've bought into the claim that BMI is a good (instead of just cheap) body composition measurement tool, it'll be almost impossible to accept a solution that fails to deliver before and after BMI data.

The Emperor's New Clothes…Right?
In other words, if you expect to see the emperor's beautiful, new clothes, you'll willingly go along with the admiring crowd instead of the young child who clearly sees the nakedness of the entire situation. If you expect to see the old hag you'll be unable to see the beautiful, young woman. And if you've bought into the status quo's experts and the media that feeds on their every syllable, it will be almost impossible for you to even entertain, let alone see a simple, natural, functional, and affordable solution like OPYOW, because it so thoroughly contradicts your expectations.

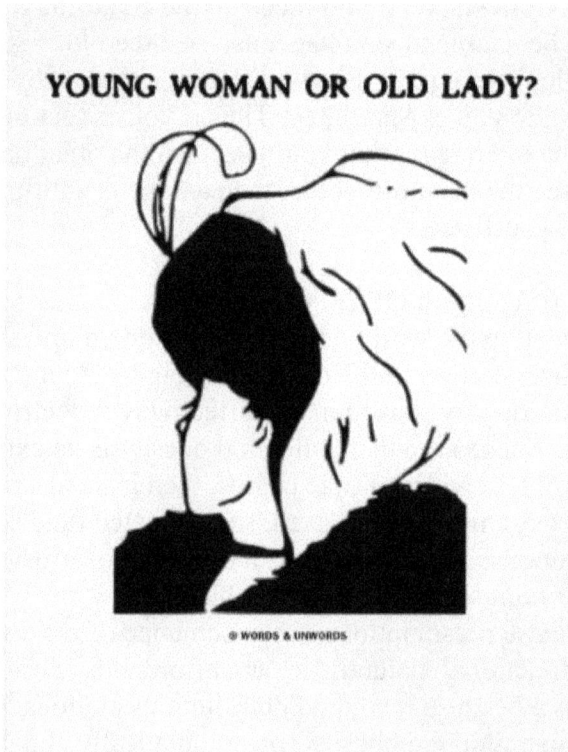

YOUNG WOMAN OR OLD LADY?

© WORDS & UNWORDS

Section 2

A Practical Solution That Kids Understand

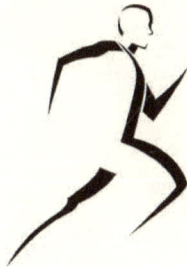

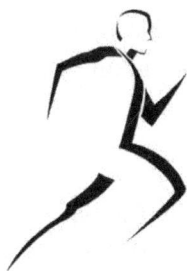

1

A Coach Offers a Solution to Childhood Obesity

Obesity is a huge problem in America and around the world. And the childhood edition of this problem is a 21st century tragedy that's not only costing our nation billions of dollars, but it's costing millions of kids their confidence, their self esteem, their willingness to try something new in public for fear of failure, and consequently their capacity to live full and productive lives.

While scientists are busy studying body chemistry, body composition, nutrition, and exercise physiology, pharmaceutical companies are busy developing the latest weight loss pill, the diet industry is designing a new diet strategies, infomercials are crowing about new exercise devices, health clubs are hustling fitness, insurance companies are cutting benefits, and McDonald's is pushing salads, all in an effort to commercially take part in the multi billion dollar obesity industry. In the mean time, the problem continues to grow unabated, like a forest fire raging out of control.

An Old Coach's Reaction

In light of that raging forest fire I'd like to introduce you to the wisdom of a retired coach who I've known for over three decades. In the words of the old coach, "I taught physical education for most of my adult life and during that time I made the following observation. I noticed that kids who could perform pull-ups were never obese," he said. "And kids who were obese could never perform pull-ups. Pull-ups and obesity are mutually exclusive, and are never found in the same kids," he added.

Without Pills, Shots, or Magic Diets

The old coach's conclusion was that if you start 'em young, before they've had a chance to pick up much weight, teach them the ability to perform pull-ups, and teach them to never lose that ability, you can immunize kids against obesity for a lifetime, without pills, shots, magic diets, or much in the way of expense. "The more kids you can teach to physically pull their own weight," he said, "the closer you'll come to whipping the childhood obesity epidemic."

But Kids Hate Pull-Ups

I told the coach that I thought his logic was impeccable, but in my view he had one problem. According to my recollection, most kids hated pull-ups with a passion. And if they hate doing it, how can you teach them to perform pull-ups? They'll drag their feet all the way to the gym, won't they?

Using a Height Adjustable Pull-Up Bar

"Kids hate doing anything where they fail in public," the coach replied. "The trick is to start them young before they learn to associate pull-ups with public humiliation. Start them out on a height adjustable bar that allows them all to succeed immediately with leg- assisted pull-ups, jumping and pulling at the same time. With this inexpensive tool you'll eliminate failure, and build regular success into the experience for all participants."

How High Do You Set The Bar

A couple more questions popped into my mind immediately. First, how high do you set the bar when you're starting a youngster out? And secondly, how do you adjust the level of difficulty in order to insure progress? I could tell however, the wise old coach had an answer on the tip of his tongue.

The Progression

"You start the bar out low enough that the child can do at least 8 leg assisted pull-ups, but no more than 12. You allow them to work out twice a week and expect them to improve every time for a number of weeks, consecutively. In other words, in the second workout they should do 9, in the third, 10, in the fourth, 11, and in the fifth, 12 leg assisted pull-ups. When they hit 12 repetitions you raise the bar one inch and they begin the 8-12 process all over again. This strategy allows a child to make a little progress every time he or she works out, and after several weeks they learn to EXPECT TO SUCCEED IN PUBLIC, which in turn teaches them to love instead of hate pull-ups."

They've Immunized Themselves Naturally

So if I understand it right Coach, the kids literally inch their way upward until they eventually run out of leg assistance, at which point they've not only learned to perform pull-ups, but they've also learned to love doing them, and in the process they've immunized themselves naturally against obesity for a lifetime as long as they maintain the ability. Does that sound about right, I asked?

They May Want To Be Bad, But

"Mechanically speaking that's correct," the coach said. But there are a few other things that go into the strategy that you need to understand. One thing is that you're tapping into a child's natural desire to be strong and not weak. In my years of teaching I met lots of kids who wanted to be bad, but I never met a kid who wants to be weak. And that goes for the boys as well as the girls. We all want to be strong. All kids know that the ability to do pull-ups requires you to be strong. And when you work in a group, they're getting stronger in public, and kids love to succeed in public," he said. "They inevitably finish off by giving each other high fives, and they love every second of it."

I asked the coach what other things are built into his strategy. He said kids learn that three things make them strong, including regular work, good eating habits, and getting enough rest at night and in between workouts. They also learn that fooling around with tobacco, alcohol, and drugs makes them weak. And no kid ever wants to be weak. "They also learn these concepts in a very hands-on, and concrete way," he said.

Taking Responsibility For Yourself

I knew the coach could have talked on this subject all day but I wanted to finish on one other related point. The phrase "Pull Your Own Weight" has responsibility taking connotations that are very appealing to most people these days. What role does taking responsibility for oneself play in this childhood obesity prevention strategy?

After congratulating me on all the good questions the old coach said, "One of the big lessons that kids learn from working on the pull-up bar is that nobody else can do it for you," he said. "I mean in reading, writing, and arithmetic you may get away with having somebody else do your homework for awhile. But the pull-up bar knows immediately if you've done the work, it knows if you're eating right, it knows if you got enough rest recently, and it pays you for doing these things with additional success.

On the other hand, it also knows if you fail to do these things, and it can just as easily deny the public success that all kids crave. So this strategy absolutely encourages kids to take responsibility for themselves in all kinds of ways," the coach said.

A Web Site Dedicated to The Old Coach's Strategy

I confessed that he'd sold me. I agreed that teaching kids to pull their own weight would go a long ways towards solving the childhood obesity epidemic, it could save our nation billions of dollars, and do all kinds of wonderful things for the individuals who learned the lessons that are built into this simple, practical, affordable, and infinitely measurable strategy. In fact I was so impressed that I offered to build an informational web site dedicated to the old coach's naturalistic vision. He took me up on the offer, and as I write this sentence you can now check out www.pullyourownweight.net if you'd like to learn more about the old coach's simple childhood obesity prevention strategy.

One Final Question

My final question to parents and educators (or anyone who works with kids) is, why wait for the experts to come up with a high tech solution when you can turn the tide naturally with your own kids right now by simply teaching them to pull their own weight? As they always say, there's no time like the present. Carpe diem.

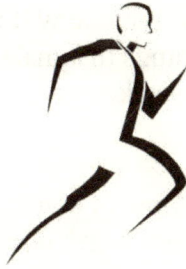

2

Two Simple Words That Motivate All Kids

Have you ever heard anyone say, "It's not so much what you say, but how you say it that counts?" As it turns out this phrase is especially true for kids.

In that light there are four words you should consider eliminating from your vocabulary when communicating with kids. They include good, bad, right, and wrong. These four words have been so effectively and successfully bastardized by the media that they no longer mean what you intend for them to mean when you're working with kids.

Now, in place of those four words, add two others that not only communicate what you want to communicate, but they motivate and activate all kids in the process. These two words are STRONG, and WEAK.

Let me say it this way. There are plenty of kids these days who take great pride in "being bad." But there's never been a kid who takes any pride in being weak at anything. Think about it. Every kid on planet Earth wants... even longs to be strong at everything. Yet not even one wants to be weak at anything.

Strong VS Weak: One Example

So for example, when explaining to Johnnie why he needs to do his math homework, try to avoid saying, "Do you want to be good or bad at math Johnnie? Instead the question should be, "Do you want to be strong or weak at math Johnnie?

In the first instance Johnnie might reply "I want to be bad," and he'll have missed your point and remain unmotivated. But you'll never hear Johnnie say "I want to be weak," because no kid wants to be weak at anything. It's un-cool to be weak. And strong is

85

always cool. In other words, Johnnie will understand and he'll make it his business to do those things that make him strong, and resist those things that make him weak.

Privilege VS Obligation

While we're on the topic of communication, there are four more words (concepts) that are worth contemplating when working with kids. They are "privilege, opportunity, obligation, and mandate." With regard to these words let me say that anything kids get to do is more valuable and more important to them than anything they have to do.

For example, if his father demands that he spend two hours a night on his homework, Joey quickly learns to see homework as an obligation not a privilege. Under these conditions his concentration and curiosity will wane, and his ability to learn will be undermined by his father's well intended, but ill conceived demands.

On the other hand if Joey understands that doing his homework makes him strong, and that most kids around the world are denied the privilege of formal education because keeping people ignorant is one way of making sure they remain weak by those who want to control them, Joey will see his homework in a completely different light. When homework is intrinsically valued, Joey's natural curiosity will blossom and maximize his concentration, his focus, and his ability to learn exponentially.

The Moral of this Story

The moral of this story is "It's not so much what you say, but how you say it that counts?" When working with kids make sure and understand the value of being strong VS being weak. And don't forget to make learning an opportunity, not an obligation.

These are small but mighty changes that can help you motivate your kids to do the things they must do in order to grow up strong, confident, and capable. In the process you'll make your job much less frustrating whether you're Joey's parent or his teacher. Joey really wants to be strong at everything and weak at nothing. Help him get there and you'll both wind up in the winner's circle.

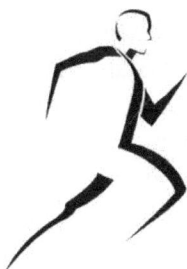

3

Abstract Generality VS Concrete Specificity in Childhood Obesity Prevention

If the NFL successfully inspired thousands of kids to play for 60 minutes a day with their Play 60 childhood obesity marketing campaign, they'll get kids to burn a lot of calories and generally move the childhood obesity debate in the right direction. If Michelle Obama succeeds with her Lets' Move campaign, and kids get moving and eating better, that too will generally move the childhood obesity debate in the right direction. If the Chicago area's CLOCC succeeds in imbedding their 5, 4, 3, 2, 1, Go mantra into the psyches of tens of thousands of young Chicagoans, and they act accordingly, it generally moves the debate in the right direction.

Moving the debate in the right direction and generally turning the tide on childhood obesity is the goal for almost every childhood obesity prevention initiative that's floating around on the market today. That includes the daily PE proponents, the get rid of the vending machine activists, and the feed 'em decent food in school lunch lines crowd. But with Operation Pull Your Own Weight we aim at a documented, concrete finality with real live individual kids in a way that nobody else can currently match.

From Abstractions to Concrete Results

In other words if you successfully set the stage for the kids in your school to learn to do pull ups, you're setting the stage for real, individual, flesh and blood kids to ELIMINATE OBESITY in their lives as soon as they cross that finish line, because kids who can do at least one pull up cannot carry 30% body fat. THEY CAN'T BE OBESE.

87

Show me ten real kids who can do at least one pull up and I'll show you ten real kids who are not obese. In other words we're not expending millions in precious, limited resources hoping to make a difference in the abstract and generally moving the debate in the right direction. OPYOW aims TO ELIMIINATE OBESITY one child, one family, one school or school district, one county, one state, and one nation at a time in a very concrete, well documented, data driven way.

Our Surveys are Qualitatively Different

In that light our surveys are not made up of the conventional "representative samplings," and reported in terms of abstract statistical gains and losses. Our surveys are made up of real schools that have real students, some of whom can do conventional, unassisted pull ups, and some of whom cannot.

So for example, if 20% of your school's students can do pull ups, you're just getting started, but the job is already 20% complete. If 50% your school's students can do pull ups, you have a year's worth of OPYOW experience under your belt and you're well on the way to winning the war on childhood obesity. If 100% of your school's students can do at least one pull up, CHILDHOOD OBESITY HAS OFFICIALLY BEEN ELIMINATED. That's the difference between infinite talk and real live action.

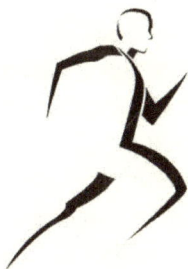

4

The Smartest, Simplest, and Cheapest Childhood Obesity Prevention Machine on Planet Earth

The two most important factors in childhood obesity plague that's haunting kids across our nation and others, are nutrition and exercise. But in a modern world that's overflowing with Big Macs, curly fries, milk shakes, soda pop, candy bars, cookies, ice cream, and sugary cereals just to mention a few, how can anyone really know for sure if their kids are falling prey to the anti-nutritional temptations that are polluting the world or fending them off?

In a world where we drive our kids to and from school instead of expecting them to walk, a world that's veritably gushing with little techno robots ranging from video games to Ipods, TV, MP3 Players to cell phones complete with a built-in video camera's designed to attract, if not demand, and command kid's attention, how does anyone make sure their kids are getting enough exercise to avoid obesity?

Complicated, Confusing, Overwhelming, Unless...

It all seems so complicated. It all seems so confusing. It all seems almost overwhelming for many parents until they recognize that there really is one extremely simple, safe, and inexpensive (dare I say cheap?) solution to the entire convoluted dilemma.

In fact you can buy one of these incredibly simple solutions at K-Mart, Wal-Mart, or Costco for as little as $10 to $15 dollars. It requires almost no space, almost no time, and being a rocket scientist is not a prerequisite for knowing how to work this little gizmo. In fact I've personally seen kindergartners handle one of these babies with the greatest of ease.

The Technical Name is...

The technical name of this wonderful little childhood-obesity-prevention-machine is a "PULL-UP-BAR." Generally speaking it's a round, chromed pipe that designed to be locked into the top of a doorway at home or in school. In fact this particular location is so common that many of these machines are actually called "DOORWAY PULL-UP-BARS."

The Trick is to Use it

Once locked into position there are no moving parts. This means the cost of upkeep on this machine is next to nothing and it's likely to last for decades, maybe more. Like most exercise equipment, the real trick with a PULL-UP-BAR is to actually use it. In other words if it becomes a dust gatherer or a clothes hanger, the odds of it preventing childhood obesity are reduced to the odds of winning the lotto, maybe worse.

How Does it Tell me What I Need to Know

"That's all well and good," you say, "but how in the world is that little PULL-UP-BAR going to tell me, any parent, or teacher whether or not a child is eating poorly or is failing to get enough exercise?" The answers to those questions are actually quite simple.

For example, let's say that you start young, helping your child learn to do pull ups when they're beginning kindergarten, and by the end of the school year they've learned to do five of them. Now, if that child starts stocking up on candy and soda pop, potato chips and pizza instead of the fruits and vegetables, they'll gain excess weight and their performance will automatically decrease.

When One Goes Up the Other Goes Down

In other words, if they eat poorly the workload (their own body weight) on the pull up bar will increase. When that happens your child's ability to perform pull ups will begin to decrease from 5 to 4 and from 4 to 3, etc. And if they eat too poorly they'll soon be unable to do any pull ups at all. In fact for years it's been common knowledge among physical educators that kids who are obese can never do pull ups, and that kids who can do pull ups are never obese.

On the other hand, if your child focuses on good eating habits, minimizes the bad stuff, and adds a little regular practice a couple times a week, they'll most likely grow stronger and their performance will increase to 6 or 7 or 8 repetitions instead of decreasing. Performance increases you see, directly reflect lower %'s of body fat, and vice versa.

The Pull Up Bar Knows

That being the case, there 's absolutely no doubt that the omniscient pull up bar knows whether your child is eating right or not, and it lets them know in no uncertain terms by increasing or decreasing their performance levels. In other words, the pull up bar pays for good eating habits with automatic performance gains. It also punishes poor eating habits with automatic performance losses. Talk about smart.

If you've read this far it won't be much of a stretch when I tell you that the exercise aspect of this scenario is very similar to the nutritional aspect. That is to say, the pull up bar pays for regular practice with automatic performance gains, and it punishes lack of practice with automatic performance losses.

Even further, the pull up bar pays for your kids to walk back and forth to school, to run and romp at recess, to play a little soccer with friends after school, because all these activities burn calories, repel excess weight, and in the end a pull up bar pays for two things. It pays for a participant to be relatively strong and light, and the feedback occurs automatically whenever you grab hold of the bar and see how many times you can physically pull your own weight.

Smarter, Simpler, Cheaper

If your performance increases, you're doing things right. If it decreases that's a sure sign that it's time to make some adjustments of your eating and/or your exercise habits. A smarter, simpler, and less expensive childhood obesity prevention machine would be extremely hard to imagine. And in this day and age, smarter, simpler, and cheaper are all wonderfully good qualities. Yes?

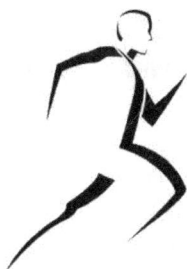

5

Three New Flavors Added to the Mix

Occasionally critics say that Operation Pull Your Own Weight is linear (i.e. incomplete, lacking well roundedness) and inflexible since it concentrates so completely on pull ups. In fact one guy went so far as to say "You'd think that pull ups are the only exercise with which you can immunize yourself against obesity for life. But I can name several exercises about which you could say exactly the same thing and it wouldn't take long for me to come up with them either."

Now it may surprise this critic, but the OPYOW team agrees with him on all counts. And in honor of this particular criticism they've decided to add three new flavors to the pull ups menu and to tell readers that they're welcome to choose any one of them in place of pull ups. And once the exercise is mastered, the participant is naturally immunized against obesity for life as long as they maintain the ability... just like pull ups.

First New Flavor - Dips

The first new flavor on the list is known simply as Dips. Generally performed on a dip station or on parallel bars, dips are similar to pull ups in that performers are handling 100% of their body weight. The dip station also automatically rewards fat loss with performance gain and it automatically punishes fat gain with performance loss... just like pull ups.

The primary difference between pull ups and dips is that they involve different sets of muscles. More specifically, pull ups (a pulling exercise) engage a participant's biceps, lats, and posterior deltoids. In contrast the dips (a pushing exercise) engage the triceps, the pecs, and the anterior deltoids.

Second New Flavor – Superman Push Ups

The second new flavor on the menu is an exercise that's known in some circles as Superman Push ups. This exercise also involves 100% of the participant's body weight, and it automatically pays for fat loss with performance gain, and punishes fat gain with performance loss, just like pull ups and dips.

But instead of biceps VS triceps, and lats VS pecs, Superman push ups primarily challenge a participant's core muscles in a way that very few exercises can match. As the result, those who can actually perform Superman push ups have abs that can withstand Kryptonite, and a six pack is all but guaranteed.

Third New Flavor

The third new addition to the OPYOW menu is an exercise known as sissy squats. Once again,100% of a participant's body weight is used, with automatic payoffs and punishments for fat loss or gain. But instead of upper body or core muscles, sissy squats concentrate on the biggest muscles in the body... your quadriceps. That's not to say that the core muscles need not stabilize throughout the range of motion. They certainly do. But the movement comes mainly from the knees... creating a body weight quad extension, so you see why these particular exercises were chosen to be the new members of the group.

Other Possibilities

Now, are there other exercises that could be mentioned in the same way? Of course there are, and they'll certainly be addressed at a later date. But for now, OPYOW participants can choose from pull ups, dips, Superman push ups, and sissy squats, which effectively quadruples the offering they've had to date. Hopefully this news clarifies OPYOW's position, and satisfies a few critics. In the meantime, what's stopping you from naturally immunizing yourself against obesity for life? Hating pull ups is suddenly a non-issue.

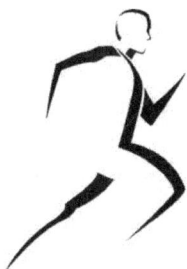

6

What About Those Kids Who Are Already Obese?

To date our comments have addressed ONLY the prevention side of the childhood obesity epidemic. But that doesn't mean we have nothing to say on the rehabilitation side. It just means that we've chosen to work on the side where the odds of winning are dramatically better by virtue of preventing the poison from ever entering the bloodstream.

You see, once the childhood obesity monster has buried its fangs into the psyche of a young boy or girl, that sucker hangs on for dear life and it grows stronger by the day, the week, the month, and the year. Breaking a bad habit is much more difficult than simply avoiding it in the first place.

We Can No Longer Sit on the Sidelines

But since there are millions of kids across the nation who are already obese, we can no longer sit on the sidelines and remain silent. However, even the rehabilitation aspect of the problem boils down to eating better and exercising more. And once this dual culprit is fully recognized, the problem can actually be boiled down to one factor...namely MOTIVATION.

In other words, you can give anyone all the right information. You can also give them access to the right tools and the right equipment. The one thing you can't give them, though, is the willpower. You can't give them the desire to take action. That is to say, you can't want it for them. If they don't want to solve the problem enough to take the necessary actions, the problem is dead on arrival and destined to remain unresolved.

The Question is...

So the real question is, how do you inspire kids who have already developed all the bad habits, and are already suffering from all the various problems that go along with being obese? How do you motivate them to give up the old "weakness producing habits" in exchange for the new, "strength producing habits?" How do you instill enough confidence for them to take the first step, leading to the second step, leading to the third step, etc.

The Answer is...

The answer to that question in our view is that someone needs to show them how to succeed immediately. Then, someone needs to help them learn to grow a little stronger, a little leaner in every workout, every week, every month, all year long. In other words, if we expect kids to invest their own time, effort, and self image into anything, those kids will expect to see a (non-monetary) tangible payoff, a dividend, a return on their investment of time and effort. And the more frequent the payoff, the higher the motivation levels will be. You can count on it.

One simple example could be, if someone goes on a diet and loses a pound/day, their motivation will be sky high. If their success is reduced to a pound/week, the motivation drops significantly. But if it's reduced to a pound/month it'll be hard to see any motivational wind in the sails. Yes, motivation is all about the frequency of success.

In Short...

In short, nothing succeeds like success. If you can deliver regular success into the lives of kids who are already obese you'll at least stand a fighting chance at turning the tide and winning the war. If not, you're wasting your time, effort, and money.

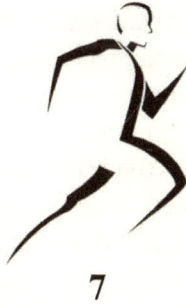

Let's Put Returning Vets to Work on Childhood Obesity Prevention

In a recent article written for the Huffington Post New York Senator Kirstin Gillibrand lamented the fact that over 20% of the troops coming home from Iraq and Afghanistan are currently unemployed. In other words these soldiers have laid their lives on the line on behalf of the USA overseas. But when they return home, the USA is unable to create jobs with which they can support themselves and their families with dignity.

In Gillibrand's words, "These days, when our troops return from Iraq and Afghanistan, so often they are coming home to a country far different than the one they left. Many of the businesses they once knew and worked at are gone. Jobs have disappeared by the millions and are only very slowly starting to return. As a result, more than 1 in 5 veterans today are unemployed. It is simply unacceptable that these hardworking, devoted men and women, who have done their job for America abroad, cannot find a new job back home."

Well Paid, Meaningful Work

In response Gillibrand has introduced a Senate bill designed to help rectify that problem. And in that same light we'd like to join the Senator when we suggest that a very high percentage of unemployed vets could easily be trained to help kids across the USA to naturally immunize themselves against obesity for life.

And once trained to combat this malignant epidemic, vets not only could, but they should be well paid for performing a valuable service in schools, park districts, YMCAs, Boys and Girls

Clubs, and other youth organizations around the nation who also want to immunize their kids against obesity for life.

Using this simple concept we can kill two problematic birds with one well placed stone. First we can reduce the unemployment among returning vets and put them in a position where they can perform meaningful work instead of the tedious meaningless work with which so many are saddled these days.

Second we can make dramatic cuts in childhood obesity, which in the long run will generate dramatic cuts in adult obesity. And while we're reducing unemployment, childhood and adult obesity, we'll simultaneously reduce the plethora of medical problems (i.e. type 2 diabetes) that are tied so directly to this 21st century epidemic.

Reducing Health Care Costs

As these two problems are cut down to size, the demand for medical services will be simultaneously reduced at the same time. And when you reduce the demand for any product or service, you automatically reduce the cost. Thus a third benefit to this strategy will be reducing the cost of healthcare nationwide. That now kills three birds with one well placed stone.

8

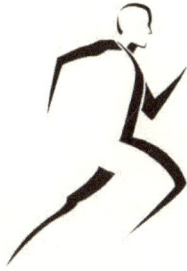

An Open Letter to Kids Around the World

Dear Kids:
I'm a former teacher who spent 17 years teaching physical education and coaching various sports. I'm also a father who has two adult age kids - to me they're still kids just like you will always be to your Mom and Dad.

Bad, but Never Weak
One way or the other, in my sixty years, I've known lots of kids and I confess that I've never met even one who wants to be weak at anything. I've met lots of kids who will tell you they want to be bad, but never one who wants to be weak. Every kid I've ever known wants to be strong (independent and adult-like) at everything and weak (dependent and child-like) at nothing, and I presume you're no exception to the rule.

Strong Kids
In that light, I've also noticed that the kids who are really strong at lots of things are also confident, and they have no need of being pretentious about much of anything. They know who they are, and they're generally happy with that.

Weak Kids
On the other hand, kids who feel like they're weak in various ways, usually lack confidence and they often feel the need to pretend to be tough, defiant, and yes BAD. These kids feel threatened by other people, especially those who are different from

99

them, and they hide behind all kinds of self erected walls and fences, including the way they dress, wear their hair, the music they listen to, and the way they interact with their parents, teachers, and peers.

The Antidote

These same kids still want to be strong at everything. But their feeling of weakness inhibits their ability to explore new possibilities because they're scared of failing and being humiliated in front of their friends. It's much safer and easier to be able to claim, "I didn't try." At least there's a viable excuse for failure, and some degree of cool is maintained. The antidote of course is to start young and help these kids learn to become strong at all kinds of things. Under these conditions the walls and fences of pretension are never erected.

A Friend?

Now let me ask you a question. If you knew an adult - a teacher or a parent - who would help you learn to become a little bit stronger every day, every week, every month, all year long, would you have lots of respect for that person? Would you be inclined to listen to that person's advice, and follow it because you know it'll make you stronger? In the long run, could an adult like this even turn out to be your friend?

Every Day, Week, Month

Let's take this conversation in a little different direction. Do you know any kids who make a practice of growing a little stronger every day, every week, every month, all year long? If someone actually did that, starting at a young age, right on into adulthood, can you imagine just how strong that person would actually become? If you did that starting at a young age, can you imagine how strong you'd be? Can you imagine how confident you'd be? Can you imagine how unique, how interesting, and how cool you'd be?

What's Important to You?

I guess the important question now is, "What's really important to you?" Given the opportunity, in what ways would you like to become strong? Would you like to have a strong body that allows you to run fast, jump high, move quickly from side to side, climb ropes, mountains, etc? Would you like to have a strong mind with which you can think, calculate, understand, read, and write creatively and productively?

Would you like to have a strong spirit that gallops to the top of the hill each morning, mane and tail flowing in the breeze, rearing up, silhouetted against the horizon in which your mind and body merge and express your admiration and appreciation to Mother Nature? God? Life?

Relentless Persistence, the Key of Keys

In order to experience life at this level, you must first recognize that you can become a little stronger every day, every week, every month, every year, for many years running. You must also recognize that you can progress regularly, if you take small bites, designed to continually reignite your motivation, resulting in a lifelong pattern of Relentless Persistence.

Finally, you must recognize that through Relentless Persistence, almost any goal can be reached by almost anyone who wants to be strong at everything and weak at nothing.

Section 3

The Supporting Data

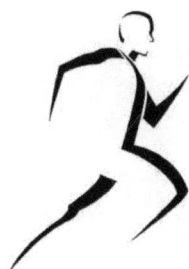

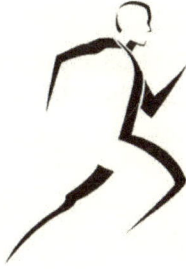

The 492 Kid Statistical Study

Hypothesis: The odds of kids who can perform at least one conventional pull up being obese are somewhere between microscopically small and non-existent.

Spring 2010
Physical Education Instructor: Debbie Larson
In conjunction with Rick Osbourne, OPYOW
Second, Third, and Fourth Graders
Galloway Elementary School, Channahon, IL
Not Peer Reviewed

Statistical Results (See Bar Graph on page 107)

• According to The US Center for Disease Control (US CDC), 17% (or 12.5 million) of all US kids between the ages of 2 and 19 are obese.

• Compare the US CDC data to the following 492 kid study containing BMI data from 290 boys and 202 girls who's ONLY qualification was, THEY COULD ALL DO AT LEAST ONE UNASSISTED PULL UP.

• Once identified, BMI scores were calculated for all 492 kids.

• As the result, according to this 492 kid study/bar graph, 0% (i.e. NONE) of the 202 GIRLS were obese, which is another way of saying, the odds were 100% AGAINST GIRLS BEING OBESE if they can do at least one pull up!

• As the result, according to this same 492 kid study/bar graph, 2% of the 290 BOYS were obese. Thus, the odds were 98% AGAINST BOYS BEING OBESE if they can do a pull up!

• Therefore, this empirical data overwhelmingly confirms the hypothesis contending that the odds of kids who can perform at least one conventional pull up being obese are somewhere between microscopically small and non-existent.

2

The Data

Summary of Children's BMI-for-Age			
	Boys	Girls	Total
Number of children assessed:	290	202	492
Underweight (< 5th %ile)	2%	1%	2%
Normal BMI (5th - 85th	83%	91%	86%
Overweight or obese (≥	14%	8%	12%
Obese (≥ 95th %ile)	2%	0%	2%

*Terminology based on: Barlow SE and the Expert Committee. Expert committee recommendations regarding the prevention, assessment, and treatment of child and adolescent overweight and obesity: summary report. Pediatrics. 2007;120 (suppl 4):s164-92.

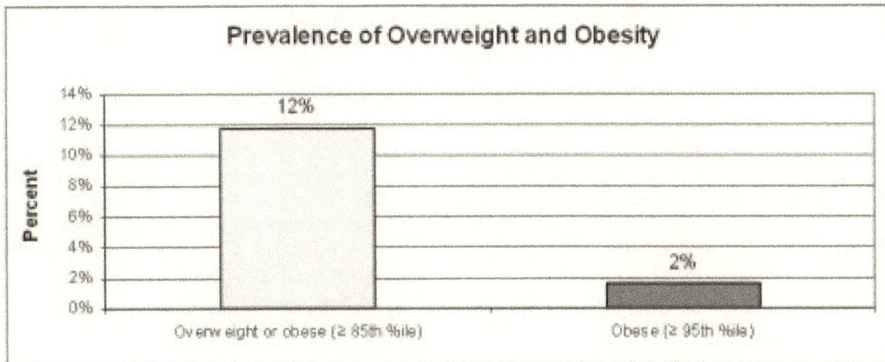

Prevalence of Overweight and Obesity

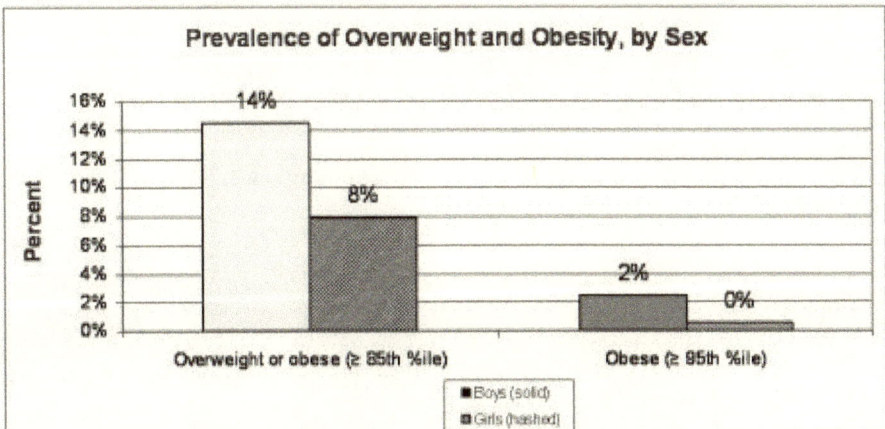

Prevalence of Overweight and Obesity, by Sex

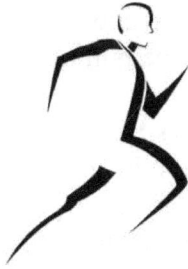

3

541 Years of P.E. Experience Confirms

Recently I was given the opportunity to make two childhood obesity prevention presentations at an event called DuPage Institute Day, the Physical Education portion of which is annually hosted by Naperville North High School in Naperville, IL. Each of my sessions attracted about 25 Physical Educators who had a particular interest in getting a handle on the childhood obesity epidemic.

During both sessions I passed around an informal survey which asked two questions. First I wanted to know how many years you'd taught PE. Second I wanted to know how many students you could recall who were both obese (i.e. 30% body fat or more) and still able to do at least one unassisted pull up. I also asked for contact information in order to substantiate the actuality of the data we gathered from the survey.

Results - 541 to 0: Worse Than Spotting Nessie

As the result of conducting this survey we had 28 out of approximately 50 attendees respond. Collectively those 28 responding Physical Educators represented 541 years worth of teaching experience. And during those 541 years worth of teaching we discovered that NOBODY could recall even one obese student who could also perform at least one conventional, unassisted pull up. In other words, the odds of spotting a student who could perform at least one pull up and still carry 30% body fat were worse than spotting Nessie or Bigfoot...0 for 541!

To extrapolate a little further yet, if each one of these teachers averaged 200 students per year (a very conservative guesstimate) it means these Physical Educators would have gone through well over 100,000 students and still never spotted even one student who could do even one pull up while carrying 30% body fat.

Educational Administrators Should be Very Interested

Now at this moment in history, when the US Surgeon General has labeled childhood obesity "America's number one health threat," this particular category of students (those who can do at least one conventional pull up) should be extremely interesting not only to Physical Educators, but to School Boards, Educational Administrators, classroom teachers, parents, and Michelle Obama herself. Why? Because according to this survey, (as well as other statistics), kids who can perform at least one conventional pull up cannot carry 30% body fat – they cannot be obese. (Test your own school district's PE teachers and see if they agree.)

Winning the War on Childhood Obesity

That being the case, winning the war on childhood obesity is simply a matter of starting kids young (kindergarten works great) and setting the stage in such a way that each student learns to physically pull their own weight. Once that goal is reached, it's a matter of eating and exercising in ways that allow them to maintain the ability to do pull ups and these students will have naturally immunized themselves against obesity and related problems for life.

In other words, if 25% of your students can do at least one unassisted pull up the job is already 25% done. When 50% can do at least one pull up, the job is half done. When 100% of your student can do at least one pull up, you will have eliminated obesity completely. You'll also have improved academic performances, and minimized anti-social behavior as well because obesity has been shown to be closely related to these other two issues. I'd call it an educational administrator's trifecta – three for the price of one.

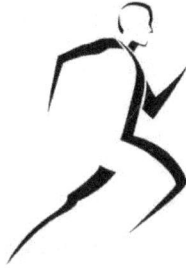

4

Insufficient Science: Oh Really?

On several occasions I've had the privilege of addressing academicians in an attempt to make the case for a functional solution to childhood obesity. Initially they agree with all my points. Then they ask for a little time to ponder the possibilities. Then more often than not they come back with some variety of the phrase "insufficient science." In other words they contend that this simple, functional solution has yet to be sufficiently tested by the academic establishment, so they withhold their support.

Ironically these are the same academicians who consistently endorse a concept known as Body Mass Index (BMI) as the preferred metric with which to measure changes in childhood obesity levels. So my reaction is "Insufficient science? Let me show you what insufficient science really looks like." Let's do a little math and see what we can discover about insufficient science.

BMI: the Formula

Body weight divided by height squared times 703 (BW/Ht squared X 703). You do recognize that as the formula for BMI, right? So in general, lose body weight and your BMI improves. On the other hand, gain body weight and your BMI deteriorates. But let's get more specific and calculate three examples in order to demonstrate the problem.

Numerical Example # 1

Let's say Bill works out real hard for 6 months and replaces 10 pounds of fat with 10 pounds of muscle mass. In this particular instance Bill's percentage of body fat has improved significantly.

His physical efficiency, his functional performance, and his metabolism have also all improved dramatically. Bill is physically better in every conceivable way – except for his BMI which has remained exactly the same because his body weight has remained exactly the same.

Numerical Example # 2

Let's try a couple of other scenarios. Bill works out real hard for six months and gains 10 pounds of muscle mass (horsepower), but didn't lose any body fat. Again, if we do the calculations, Bill's percentage of body fat improves, his physical efficiency, his functional performance, and his metabolism all improve, yet his BMI has deteriorated significantly because his body weight increased by 10 pounds.

Numerical Example # 3

How about one more scenario to drive the point home? Let's say that Bill gets sick and loses 10 pounds of muscle mass (horsepower). In this case Bill's percentage of body fat, his physical efficiency, his functional performance, and metabolism have all deteriorated significantly. But lo and behold, his BMI has improved significantly because Bill lost 10 pounds of body weight. From these three examples it's easy to see that BMI (on its own) is completely unable to distinguish between a 6 foot, 200 pound block of granite and a 6 foot, 200 pound mold of Jello.

Individuals VS the Masses

In the face of this kind of unarguable evidence these high minded, empirically oriented, data driven academicians usually relent and confess that BMI is probably not the best metric for individuals. On the other hand they contend, for large groups of people, BMI is still a valid metric.

That's Insufficient Science in Spades

At that point, anyone who's listening closely will be forced to ask, "What is a large group of people if not a collection of individuals?" So, if BMI is invalid for individuals, how does it suddenly become valid for a collection of individuals?

Any way you slice it, if you really want to see what insufficient science looks like, all that's required is to seriously consider the merits of BMI and you'll find it in spades. You won't please the guardians of the status quo, but you'll get a real good taste of insufficient science. The functional solution however, is quite another story. If you're interested resolving childhood obesity you might want to check it out.

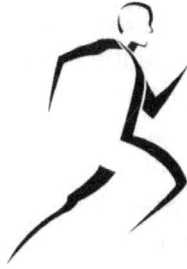

5

Prove It! Show Me the Evidence.

Obese kids are unable to do lots of things that kids of normal weight can do, and one of those things is conventional pull ups. In that light, one very simple solution to childhood obesity is to help all kids learn to do pull ups, (it's easy to do) because the odds of kids who can do even one pull up being obese are remote at best. And if they eat and exercise in ways that allow them to maintain the ability, the odds of them ever being obese are equally remote.

But in the process of introducing this simple solution to this complex, expensive problem, I can't tell you how many times I've had people say, "Prove it. Show me the evidence." The following represents an effort to prove this contention on three different levels.

The Big Foot Logic Test

The first level of proof is what I call the Big Foot Logic Test, and I give this test whenever I address a group of people on the topic of childhood obesity prevention. First I ask how many people in the group have ever seen Big Foot. Next I ask how many have seen the Loch Ness Monster (Nessie). And finally I ask how many have ever seen an obese person who can do even one pull up. The odds of anyone raising their hand are precisely the same in all three cases.

What this little experiment proves is the contention that "obese people are unable to do pull ups" is intuitively obvious to anyone who seriously considers the possibility. In other words, our own real life experiences support the contention. It's as plain as the nose on your face.

The second part of the Big Foot Logic Test is a simple exercise in logic. That is to say, if you agree that obese people are unable to do pull ups, you're automatically inferring that people who can do pull ups are not obese.* Logically speaking, it's impossible to agree with one statement without agreeing with the other. They're flip sides of the same logical coin.

Statistical Test # One

The second level of proof is for those empirically oriented, data driven scientists who doubt their own intuition along with the validity of their own logic. In other words, unless a contention is supported by data and statistics, this group remains skeptical.

In this light we point to a statistical study that included 492 kids (second, third, and fourth graders) whose only qualification was that everyone in this group could do at least one conventional pull up. Once this group was identified, BMI scores were run on each participant. Of the 202 girls who participated, ZERO PERCENT had BMI's of 30 or higher. Of the 290 boys who participated, 2% had BMI's of 30 or higher – 98% had BMI's of less than 30! Thus from a statistical perspective our contention is still bullet proof and irrefutable.

We readily admit that to date this statistical study lacks a university letterhead. It also lacks vetting and peer review by the medical establishment. And it has yet to be published in an officially recognized medical journal. But we're also quick to point out that this is no major obstacle since the study is so easy to duplicate...if you're willing to invest an hour or two of time and effort.

Do it Yourself Data...

On this level you start by disregarding everything we've said so far. Then go to the Physical Education Department of your local school district, identify 10 boys and 10 girls who can do at least one conventional pull up, and record their height, body weight, birth date, and gender. With that info in hand, run BMI scores on all 20 kids and see if any one of them have BMI scores of 30 or more. As you already suspect, odds are all 20 kids will have BMI scores of below 30.

By virtue of participating in this final level you'll generate your own data, your own statistics (free of anyone's prejudices), not to mention your own intuition and your own logic. Then, if you use your own self-generated data to systematically help increase the percentage of kids who can physically pull their own weight, you'll be taking one giant step towards beating childhood obesity in your community. In the words of Gandhi, "Action exposes priorities."

*This actually needs to be stated in terms of odds instead of absolutes. For example we should say, "The odds of an obese person doing pull ups are remote. Thus the odds of a person who can do pull ups being obese are equally remote.

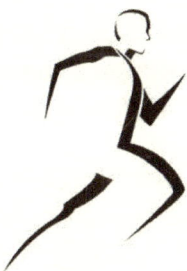

6

Data From Six Childhood Obesity Solutions

In the hyper-scientific, results-oriented, data-driven world of academia everyone claims to bow down to the numbers, the hard, cold, empirical facts. But in the world of childhood obesity prevention it's insightful to throw a spotlight on exactly what some of the experts mean when they talk on and on about their hard, cold, empirical facts.

In that light we decided to focus on the ACTUAL RESULTS (copied word for word from their respective websites) of six childhood obesity prevention interventions. Five of these are affiliated with large, well known bureaucracies including BCBS of Massachusetts, The American Academy of Pediatrics, Children's Memorial Hospital of Chicago, and the National Dairy Council. They're also financially supported by numerous well-heeled corporate partners and the federal government. The sixth is small and actively operating in only a few DuPage County (northern IL) communities. Check them all out and see what you think.

RESULTS (BCBS of Massachusetts) 5-2-1-0

Most administrators and teachers, and half of the parents reported being more aware of the 5-2-1-0 message as a result of the project. Eighty percent of the teachers who reported using the resource kit found it easy or extremely easy to use. Ninety percent of the teachers reported that they would be willing to continue implementing strategies in the future; of those who would not, a lack of time was cited as the reason. All administrators reported that the project had been worthwhile for their district.

Parents were less aware of the message than teachers and administrators; 2 in 5 parents reported receiving educational

119

handouts. Most students responded positively to the messages. (Portland, Main spent $3.7 million dollars on 5-2-1-0 over five years and it's worth checking out their hard, cold, data-driven results.)

RESULTS (Children's Memorial/Chicago) 5-4-3-2-1-GO:
Parents who received counseling consumed more fruits and vegetables at follow-up (OR 1.749, [95% CI: 1.01-3.059]). Parental exposure to messaging at children's school events was associated with higher water consumption (6.879, [1.954-24.212]).

RESULTS :Action for Healthy Kids
Action for Healthy Kids is the nation's leading non-profit and largest volunteer network fighting childhood obesity and undernourishment by partnering with schools to improve nutrition and physical activity to help our kids learn to eat right, be active every day, and be ready to learn. The Illinois Action for Healthy Kids Team (for example) is committed to increasing its work directly with schools and districts in 2009-10 by building its membership and utilizing proven programs that generate excitement about healthy schools.

In 2008-09, the Illinois Team (for example):
•Worked with more than 100 districts across Illinois.
•Helped schools in Decatur promote physical activity through activity paths, fitness centers, and other school programming.
•Convened the second Illinois School Wellness Conference, in conjunction with the Illinois State Board of Education, attracting 150 school nutrition and physical activity professionals.

RESULTS Fuel Up to Play 60:
Fuel Up to Play 60 is making a positive mark on schools and students all across the country. This year's Challenges are helping kids interact creatively with the program while adopting healthy eating habits and getting in 60 minutes of physical activity a day. (If you click the above link you'll see they also claim to be in 66% of schools across the nation, while working with 300,000 kids.)

RESULTS PE 4 Life: PE4life

Core Principles provide a platform for a variety of health and wellness activities as well as collaborative opportunities for increasing socially responsible behaviors. Research has shown a strong correlation between fitness scores, academic performance, behavior and attendance in students. PE4life works towards helping schools positively impact children's fitness levels using a variety of strategies to get kids more active.

Data collected from programs we've worked with by research universities demonstrates increased fitness levels. In addition to this, some schools that have integrated PE4life's Core Principles have shown improvements in academic performance and others have shown decreased discipline incidents. These measurable outcomes have gained the attention of business, foundation, school and community leaders who have since come together to use PE4life as a platform for collaboration.

RESULTS: OPERATION PULL YOUR OWN WEIGHT:

Out of 492 students (202 girls and 290 boys, second, third, and fourth graders attending Galloway Elementary in Channahon, IL) all of whom were able to do at least one conventional, unassisted pull up, NONE OF THE GIRLS fell into the obese category, while 2% of the boys did – 98% however DID NOT.

And since it's been shown that there's a 3% margin of error in all conventional body composition measurement tools, it's arguable that the 2% figure for boys was actually a function of the accuracy problems inherent in Body Mass Index which was the measurement tool used in this survey.

In other words, it's likely that NONE OF THE BOYS fell into the obese category either. Conclusion? Help your kids learn to do pull ups and they'll have naturally immunized themselves against obesity. Translated that means if they can do at least one pull up, odds are they can't carry 30% body fat.

The Question Now Becomes...

After reading and considering all these "bottom line results," the question becomes which of these six interventions look like they have any genuine cold, hard, empirical data to substantiate their continued existence and potential success? If you really were a results-oriented, data-driven, charitable foundation, which of these interventions would you be most interested in supporting, endorsing, implementing, and generally being affiliated with? And most importantly, which of these interventions would you recommend to your own kids or grandkids? The choice looks simple doesn't it?

Section 4

Basic Mechanics of Operation Pull Your Own Weight

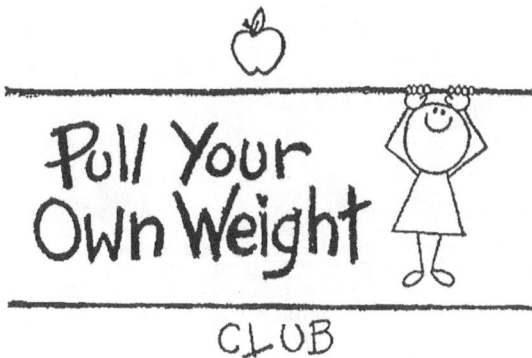

Pull Your Own Weight

CLUB

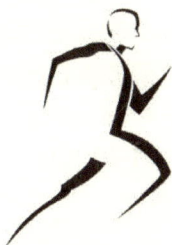

1

The Mechanics of OPYOW
(Leg Assisted Pull-ups on
Height Adjustable Pull-up Straps)

1. Attach straps/grips to any pull-up bar in any gym.

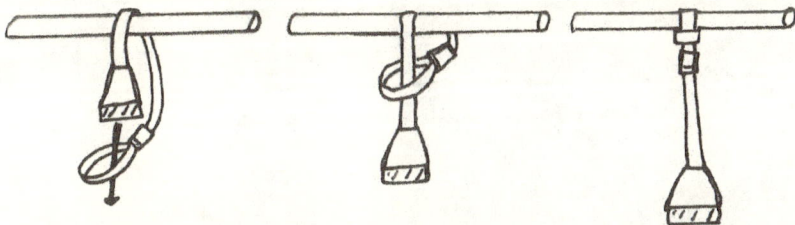

1. Place handle over pull up bar

2. Thread handle and strap through attachment loop.

3. Pull tight to secure straps.

2. Adjust the grip's height to a level where the student feet are on the floor and they can EASILY perform 9 leg assisted pull-ups (jumping/pulling simultaneously).

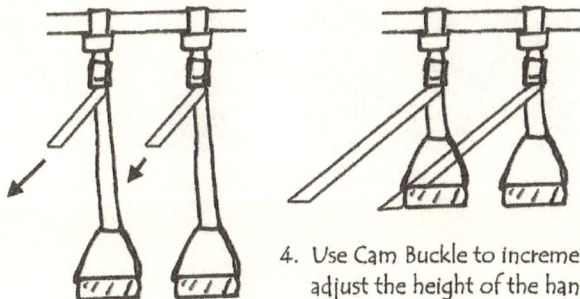

4. Use Cam Buckle to incrementaly adjust the height of the handles

125

3. Allow the student to perform 9 leg assisted pull-ups (all the way up - chin touching the grips, and all the way down - feet touching the floor), and designate it as workout # 1.

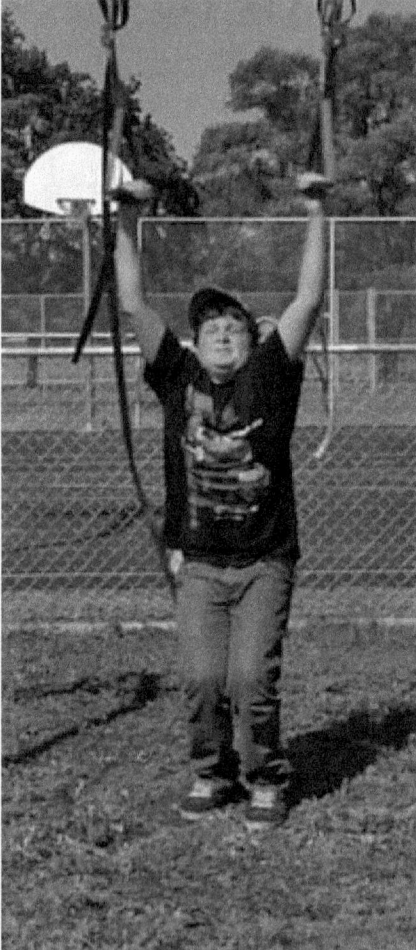

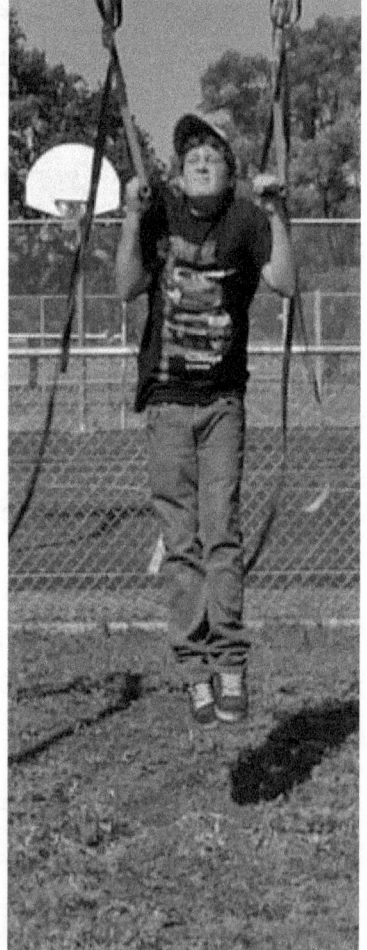

4. DOCUMENT it on the OPYOW Progress Chart

OPYOW 10 Week Sample Progress Chart

Name _____

Start Date_____

Week/Date	Level (in Inches)	Reps/Progress
Wk 1/		9
Wk 1/		10
Wk 2/		11
Wk 2/		12
Wk 3/		9
Wk 3/		10
Wk 4/		11
Wk 4/		12
Wk 5/		9
Wk 5/		10
Wk 6/		11
Wk 6/		12
Wk 7/		9
Wk 7/		10
Wk 8/		11
Wk 8/		12
Wk 9/		9
Wk 9/		10
Wk 10/		11
Wk 10/		12

REMEMBER…2 Workouts Per Week

AND YOUR GOALS ARE TO GROW:
- A Little Stronger This Week Than Last!
- A Little Stronger This Month Than Last!
- A Lot Stronger This Year Than Last!

5. We suggest students should do 2 workouts per week, on NON-CONSECUTIVE days, i.e. Mon/Thurs, Tues/Fri).

6. Workout # 2 the student performs 10 leg assisted pull-ups.

7. Workout # 3 the student performs 11 leg assisted pull-ups.

8. Workout # 4 the student performs 12 leg assisted pull-ups.

10. DOCUMENT each and every workout on the student's OPYOW Progress Chart.

11. In Workout # 5 (starting in week 3) THE GRIPS ARE RAISED ONE INCH, and the entire 9 to 12 routine is repeated all over again for 4 more consecutive workouts (2 more weeks).

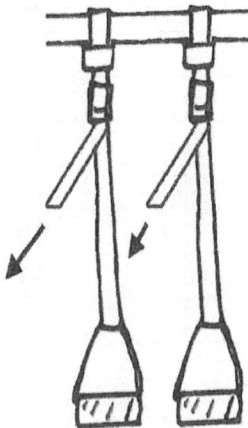

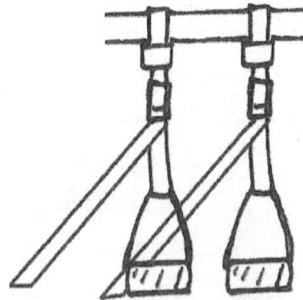

4. Use Cam Buckle to incrementaly adjust the height of the handles

12. So for example, every 2 weeks (4 workouts) the grips should be raised one inch. That means in 10 weeks, the grips will have been raised FIVE INCHES, and the student will have experienced documented progress in 20 consecutive workouts in front of their peers, along with the high fives, and confidence that accompanies it. They will also learn to look forward to each new opportunity to get on the grips (bar) and to get stronger, in front of their friends, because succeeding in public is FUN! Success, breeds success.

13. Experiencing very small, but consistent increments of progress, over an extended period of time encourages high levels of motivation, which translates into persistence. Eventually the student will run out of leg assistance, at which point they're able to do conventional pull-ups and will have naturally immunized themselves against obesity for life, as long as they maintain the ability to do pull-ups.

14. The only thing left now is to START NOW! Procrastination is the opposite of ACTION!

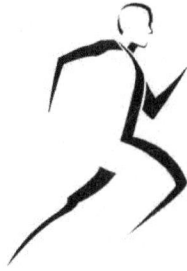

2

Avoiding the Two Big Mistakes in Functional Childhood Obesity Prevention

There are two mistakes to avoid in Operation Pull Your Own Weight (OPYOW). Mistake number one is making the starting point too difficult. And mistake number two is attempting to progress in large chunks instead of small, but regular increments over time.

The long term goal of OPYOW is to help kids naturally immunize themselves against obesity for life by learning and maintaining the ability to physically pull their own weight, i.e. to perform pull ups. The short term goal of OPYOW is to motivate participants enough to help them persist until they successfully cross the finish line.

Cultivating Motivational Momentum

So in terms of the short term goal, the strategy is to cultivate a pattern of success (what we like to call motivational momentum) in which kids learn to expect success instead of failure. Furthermore we want their peers to expect each participant to succeed instead of fail as well.

When everyone in the room is expecting success instead of failure, including and especially the participants themselves, the tendency is to dig a little deeper in order to give it 110%. When that happens, the odds of success grow exponentially.

It's Almost Impossible to...

In this light the reader will understand when I say that it's almost impossible to make the starting point too easy. It's also almost impossible to make the increments of progress too small.

If the starting point is easy and the increments are small but regular, and carried out over time, success becomes almost inevitable. And in the process participants will avoid injuries that crop up when the intensity is too great and the pushing is too hard. Also, in the process they will avoid losing motivational momentum because their investment of time and effort is continually yielding small but regular returns.

To finish off with the proverbial cliché, there's an old saying that goes, "Inch by inch success is a cinch. And Yard y yard success is hard. Remember this when learning to pull your own weight.

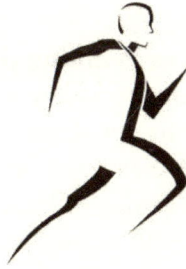

3

Cultivating a Strong Functional Immune System Prevents Childhood Obesity

Creating new antibodies (white blood cells) through the process of vaccination is how kids are systematically immunized against polio, diphtheria, small pox, and measles. Creating new functional antibodies through the process of functional childhood obesity prevention is how 21st century kids can systematically immunize themselves against today's # 1 health threat, childhood obesity. Check it out.

Step One...

Step one is to frame childhood obesity in terms of a physical disability that requires preventative action BEFORE the disability actually strikes. You don't wait until your kids get polio before vaccinating them, right? Childhood obesity requires/demands the same preventative foresight if we're going to have any chance of winning this war that's being waged against kids throughout the developed world.

What Does it Look Like?

How do you do that? And what do functional obesity antibodies look like? It's actually quite simple. Functional obesity antibodies look like conventional pull ups, conventional bar dips, rope climbing, hand stand push ups, or single legged squats.

Odds are About the Same as Winning the Lottery

Simply stated, the odds of kids who can perform even one repetition of conventional pull ups (bar dips, hand stand push ups, etc.) being obese are about the same as winning the lottery or getting struck by lightening. And the odds of kids who can perform 5 or 10 repetitions being obese are even worse because they have 5 to 10 times the functional antibodies at work on their behalf.

The Obesity Industrial Complex has Undermined Kids

The problem is that in the 21st century the bad guys (collectively known as the Obesity Industrial Complex) have successfully undermined our kid's functional immune systems to the point that most kids (80% or more) are unable to perform any pull ups, bar dips, or rope climbs. The good news however is that if they're given access to the right experiences, most kids (95% or more) can easily develop plenty of functional obesity antibodies, and in the process they naturally immunize themselves against the toxic influences that stalk them every hour of every day, week in and week out.

One Example…

Let's explore one example of how kids can actively cultivate functional obesity antibodies and in the process immunize themselves against these omnipresent influences. By using a combination of height adjustable pull up straps and a technique called leg assisted pull ups (jumping and pulling at the same time) all kids can find a place to begin successfully, and to progress regularly until they've finally conquered the functional mountain known as pull ups.

Some kids will complete the task in 6 weeks. Others will require 6 months or even more. But in the end, if they persist and are motivated by successfully making small but regular increments of progress, they will eventually cross the finish line. And as long as they maintain the ability to perform at least one conventional pull up, they will actively avoid the 21st century obesity trap for life. It's about that simple.

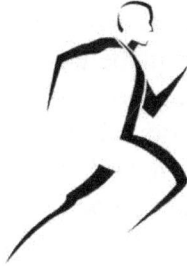

4

Our Basic Position on Nutrition: H = N/C

Operation Pull Your Own Weight is occasionally criticized for failing to spend enough time and energy on the nutritional side of the childhood obesity equation. Historically we've encouraged the kids we work with to choose "strong foods" (i.e. fruits and veggies) over "weak foods" (i.e. pizza and curly fries), presuming that kids understand this language and are motivated by the prospect of becoming stronger with their friends.

Without undermining this basic stance in any way however, we'd like to dig into the nutritional side a little deeper and become more specific on what we mean by strong foods VS weak foods. Check it out.

The Formula, H = N/C

While reading the book entitled Eat to Live by Dr. Joel Fuhrman I discovered a simple formula that serves our purposes completely and totally. The formula reads H = N/C which translates as Health Equals Nutrition Divided by Calories.

Dr. Fuhrman's basic position here is that the human body runs on nutrition much like a car runs on gasoline, or a Mack Truck runs on diesel fuel. In other words, we need nutrition in order to function. A body out of nutrition is like a car out of gas/fuel.

Strong VS Weak Foods

Furthermore, nutrition comes in the form of energy packages known as calories. Some calories are overflowing with nutrition (strong foods). Other calories contain some nutrition (average foods). And some calories contain very little nutrition (weak foods).

From a nutritional perspective the problem is that a modern, 21st century diet is too often made up of relatively empty calories – nutritionally deficient, weak foods. So in order to get enough nutrition, we end up eating lots of nutritionally deficient calories. Couple that phenomenon with modern sedentary lifestyles and you have the makings of a first class epidemic on your hands.

Nutritionally Dense Food Without Lots of Calories

All that said, making an effort to fill up on nutritionally dense (strong) foods like spinach, broccoli, kale, and collard greens, allows you to fill up on nutrition without piling up lots of calories. Let me say this in a little different way because it's really important. You can fill up on nutrition (that your body requires) without filling up on calories. The result is, your hunger is gone, you're loaded with nutrition, and your body naturally becomes stronger, lighter, and more capable of handling the active requirements of living whether athletic or academic.

Hats Off to Dr. Fuhrman

In that light I'd like to say hats off to Dr. Joel Fuhrman and his magical formula that tells you everything you need to know about nutrition. Add that information to the functional explanation that we've been discussing for some time now and you'll be living life on a higher plane. Just remember, H = N/C and eat accordingly.

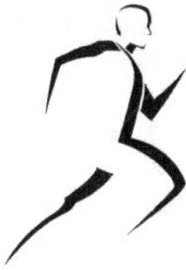

5

Strong Table, Weak Table: A School Experiment

Picture a school cafeteria at high noon, with kids streaming through, carrying their omnipresent backpacks, books, and chatting away with friends as they approach the school food court. When they arrive they suddenly notice there are now two lines instead of one. Over the top of line one is posted a big green sign that reads "STRONG FOODS." Over the top of line two is posted a big red sign that reads "WEAK FOODS."

Strong Food VS Weak Food

In the first line kids see fresh fruits and vegetables, along with low fat dairy products, whole grain breads and pasta, nuts, along with small portions of fish and fowl, etc. In the second line kids see the conventional burgers, fries, chips, pizza, sugary drinks, candy bars, etc. Then they realize that they must choose between line one and line two.

How Long Will it Take

Let's point out that there's an experiment going on here. It's designed to answer the question, "How long will it take for the weak food's demand to decrease to a point that it's no longer financially viable for the school to carry it? In other words, how long will it take the strong foods to eliminate the weak foods from the school cafeteria altogether just by virtue of hanging up a couple of signs, and by separating the good food apart from the garbage?"

They're Laying Their Bets

The administrators have taken bets on the question. Some are predicting two weeks, while others think that it will take the better part of a month before the kids will avoid the weak foods like the plague and begin embracing the strong foods instead. "After all," one administrator said, "not one kid on planet Earth wants to be weak at anything. They all want to be strong at everything because strong is cool."

Huntington, WV or Your Town, USA

So how long do you think it will take? And maybe the place to conduct this experiment is Huntington, WV where Jamie Oliver tried revolutionize school cafeteria food last year. Maybe it should be in Washington, DC right under Congress' long and condescending nose. Or maybe the place to start is Your Town, USA. I mean, every town has a school cafeteria, right? And anyone can make up a couple of signs, and separate the good and the bad food right?

My own bet is that this simple experiment will not only kill the problem of bad food inside the school walls, but it will also cause students to see food in a different light when they're outside the school walls as well. Strong food VS weak food is pretty simple. Kids will understand that real fast. Why not give it a try?

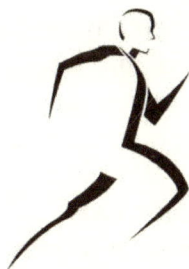

6

Like Your Kids, Rufus is a Natural Born Runner

Rufus is a dog who loves to run. He's a snow white, 28 lb. Jack Russell Terrier who's so full of energy that he's hard to appreciate without seeing him in action. He spends a good percentage of his life suspended in mid-air (some call it levitation) in between vertical leaps (some call it Michael Jordan) that lifts him eyeball to eyeball with his humans.

But given the opportunity, Rufus is so affectionate that he'll lick your face off. He also loves to chase squirrels and cars, which is why he's leashed when we go out to take care of official business.

Rufus loves running free

On good weather days Rufus spends time at the park in back of an elementary school where there are several acres with no streets for him to dash into, and no cars for him to chase after. In that setting the Rufmeister is unleashed and allowed to do what he loves to do…run freely. His coloring helps to spot him at a distance. He also comes when called, so safety is a non-issue.

Once off the leash Rufus runs at various speeds, stops and sniffs some tantalizing tidbits, and then he takes off running again. And once in a while Rufus meets other dogs in the neighborhood there. The fun these dogs have running, chasing, sniffing, tumbling all over each other is a sight to behold.

Rufus was not taught to love running…

Now…one quick observation. Rufus was not taught to love running. Loving to run came naturally, as with all dogs. Sure, there are the occasional, overly domesticated dogs who are fat and waddle from place to place. But they're probably older, and have

139

undoubtedly spent most of their days inside, lying around in front of the TV snoozing. However, if you start 'em young, and give 'em the opportunity to develop naturally, it's perfectly normal for dogs to love running and romping… just like your kids love it.

It's in his genes, just like your kids…
Learning to run follows in sequence just after learning to walk. Once walking is mastered, dogs and kids automatically want to speed up, which is when running is first experienced. Think about this. Have you ever seen the look of sheer ecstasy on a child's face at the moment they realize they're walking…and then again when they realize they're running? And when other kids show up to play, the feeling of ecstasy is amplified while they run and romp just like Rufus and Tigger in back of the school.

Kids must first be safe before you unleash them. But if that ecstasy they experience when first learning to walk and run is carefully cultivated over weeks and months for the first several years of their life, you'll find that your kids will gradually increase their love of running. As a natural byproduct, they'll also burn plenty of calories, develop good muscles, hearts, and lungs, have lots of fun, and eliminate stress, all without you having to teach anything. Given the opportunity, they'll learn on their own.

The Big Mistake
In fact the big mistake is when adults try to teach kids to run. Kids are pitted against one another creating winners and losers. Or they're encouraged to run around and around some school yard marathon style, bored to tears, and more winners and losers are created. And worst of all is when the gym teacher, a.k.a. the local high school football coach, uses running as punishment. "Give me two laps you slacker." Sound familiar? A better way to undermine anyone's natural love of running is hard to imagine.

The bureaucracy is incredibly good at taking something that's an opportunity (I get to run) and transforming it into an obligation (I have to run), while sucking out every ounce of joy and fun, and turning it into sheer drudgery. Is it any wonder that our kids are getting fatter by the second? The big question becomes how do we correct our mistakes?

140

Let Them Run, Don't Make Them Run

The first part of that correction is to begin to see running (or anything else you want a child to learn) as a privilege, as something they get to do instead of an obligation, something they have to do. The second part is to relentlessly cultivate that natural desire by giving your kids the opportunity to expand on their initial experience (i.e. to learn more) safely, and celebrate every little improvement they make.

Given that opportunity and related support, they'll naturally learn to be a little better this week than they were last, a little better this month than last, and a lot better this year than last. Given the opportunity, that's how kids grow naturally.

In other words, give them the opportunity to learn what you want them to learn (running in this case) and you'll have to teach them very little. They'll experiment and soak up their experiences like the natural born sponges that they are. So if you let them learn, and avoid forcing them to learn, you'll be amazed at how much your kids will pick up naturally, and how little you'll have to teach them.

Section 5

Motivational Psychology

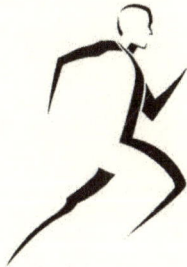

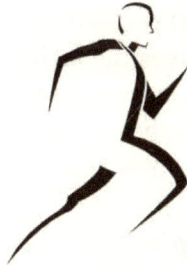

1

Motivating Kids to Eat Better and Exercise More

Multifaceted, complicated, and confusing are the kind of terms most experts currently use to describe the 21st Century childhood obesity dilemma. Arguably there are genetic, environmental, economic, sociological, and psychological factors that play a role in an issue the Attorney General of the United States has recently called "an epidemic, a pandemic, and a terrorist threat from within."

A Two Factor Dilemma...

On the other hand, when reality bashes in the door, all these complications can easily be boiled down to two factors that we all understand. They are exercise and nutritional habits. In other words, there's not one American child who can't beat obesity by sufficiently raising their physical activity level and eating less/better.

Boiled Down to One Basic Challenge...

Childhood obesity prevention then can be boiled down to one basic challenge. Namely, how can we motivate kids exercise more and eat less/better? The fact is, even if their genes, environment, economics, social network or their psychological state make it harder for some children, any child who exercises enough and eats right will successfully avoid the 21st Century obesity trap.

And One Answer

That being the case, what motivates kids? The answer is, success always breeds success, and kids are no exception to this rule. Like an investor who experiences regular returns on his financial investment, kids who experience documented returns (in the form of regular progress) on their investments of time and effort, are motivated to continue investing as long as it continues to pay off. Consistently high levels of motivation translate into persistence. And relentless persistence is the key to success in anything, including childhood obesity prevention.

Let's Focus on One Example

Pull-ups for example, are very challenging for most kids today and they're impossible for kids who carry much excess weight because of the increased workload. But, if a bar is lowered to the point where the kid's feet are flat on the floor, there are very few kids who are unable to jump and pull themselves (their chins) up to the bar. This simple technique is known as leg assisted pull-ups.

Inching Your Way Up

More specifically the strategy is to lower the bar to a level where a participant can easily do 8 leg assisted pull-ups, and allow them do a set of 8 reps. Working two days a week, say Mondays and Thursdays, the child comes back on day two (Thursday) and you allow them to do 9 leg assisted pull-ups. (1) In workout number three you allow them to do 10, in workout number four they do 11, in workout number five they do 12, and in workout number six the bar is raised one inch and the entire 8 to 12 routine is repeated all over, again and again until the child has run out of leg assistance and has mastered the ability to do conventional pull-ups.

Small Increments of Change

What I'd like to point out in this example is the extremely small increments of change, that underwrite the extremely regular experience of progress, that translates into consistently high levels of motivation, that eventually leads to relentless persistence and eventual success at anything, including the ability to do pull-ups.

Success Magnified

The value of this experience in success can be magnified even further by conducting the activity in a social setting with other kids participating too. Then as kids make predictable progress workout after workout, week after week, month after month, their success is recognized and celebrated immediately with high fives from fellow participants and teachers who are supervising. It doesn't take long for kids to realize that successfully tackling a difficult task in public is fun and they soon begin to look forward to their next opportunity to get stronger on the pull up bar.

Motivation Embedded Into the Genetic Fabric

And as any gym teacher will attest, once any child has mastered pull-ups, they're naturally immunized against obesity for life as long as they maintain the ability, because people who can do pull-ups are never obese.

But in the process, it's all about 3 things, motivation, motivation, and motivation. And the key to that vault is small, but regular increments of success, day after day, week after week, that over time, accumulate like compound interest in a bank and embeds the mantra "Oh Yes I Can" deep into the genetic fabric of any kid who's exposed to this life altering experience. May they all be exposed to this kind life altering experience at an early age.

(1) To be completely clear. The kids are allowed only 2 workouts per week. They're allowed to do only the number of pull-ups that are expected during that particular workout. Done this way you can insure that your kids experience progress (winning) every time they touch the bar for weeks and weeks in front of their friends and teacher. Under these conditions it doesn't take long before your kids are begging for the opportunity to do more pull ups. Warning, avoid giving in if you really want to keep those motivational flames burning brightly for a long, long time.

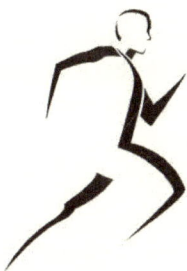

2

The Seven Motivational Pistons of OPYOW

In OPYOW there are seven motivational pistons* that blend, weave, and synergistically work together in order to motivate kids to relentlessly persist until they've learned to physically pull their own weight, and naturally immunize themselves against obesity for life.

Piston # 1: Strong at Everything

First, there is the natural desire of all kids to be strong at everything and weak at nothing. Strong is always cool, while weak is always un-cool (humiliating). You'll find kids who take pride in "being bad," but none who take pride in "being weak" at anything. It's about dignity and self respect. So, we substitute the terms Strong and Weak in place of the terms Good and Bad whenever possible. In the process we take full motivational advantage of this natural predisposition that's imbedded into the DNA of all kids.

Piston # 2: Opportunity/Privilege VS Obligation/Mandate

Second, anything that's perceived as an opportunity (I get to do it) is inevitably valued more highly than anything that's perceived as an obligation (I have to do it). So we go to great lengths to present OPYOW as an opportunity instead of an obligation.

More specifically, no one is ever forced to participate. They all get to participate because they choose to do so. When we start counting reps in workout number one, the participant gets to do 8 reps, not 9 or 10. In workout number two they get to do 9 reps not 10 or 11, etc.

If you use the right language and present the strategy in the right light, the kids will begin to look forward to the opportunity to get on the bar and get strong along with the rest of their friends. We never forget, an opportunity is always more valuable than an obligation, and it's OPYOW's second big motivator.

Piston # 3: Creating a Class Full of Winners

Third, we are staunch proponents of self competition. We want to see Johnny this week competing with Johnny last week, Johnny this month with Johnny last month. We don't want to see Johnny competing with Jimmy, or Sally competing with Susie.

In fact OPYOW defines winning as being a little stronger this week than you were last week, a little stronger this month than you were last month, and a lot stronger this year than you were last year. In this way we can create a class full of WINNERS instead of a few winners, a bunch of average participants, and a handful of LOSERS. Because winning is an extremely potent motivator, in OPYOW we make it a point to avoid creating losers/humiliation.

Piston # 4: We Measure and Document Weekly

Fourth, any time you measure anything, you're implying that it's important for some reason. And the more frequently you measure it, the more important that thing becomes. Studies have shown that doing nothing more than measuring something on a regular basis causes that thing to improve. In OPYOW we measure each kid's pull up progress twice a week (instead of the conventional once a quarter or once a semester with BMI) which makes it real important and therefore REAL MOTIVATING.

Piston # 5: Regular Success

Fifth, nothing succeeds like success. In OPYOW we set the stage in such a way that the starting point for each child is EASY, and we're assured of success. Furthermore, the increments of progress are very small, which insures regular success week after week, and month after month, all year long. In this light, success becomes a habit and kids begin to expect success (winning) instead of failure (losing) every time they grab hold of the grips. And when the going gets tough, which it always does, they dig in even harder in order to continue their success/winning, because as we said previously, winning always feels good.

Piston # 6: Winning In Public

The sixth factor is that we always do the OPYOW workouts in public, in front of peers, friends, and teachers. Because of this, every time the child lets go of the grips he/she succeeds, gets high fives from their pals and pats on the backs from the teacher. They quickly learn that tackling a difficult task like pull ups, in public is fun…as long as you succeed…which they do. The public character of the experience magnifies the successes exponentially.

Piston # 7: Tangible and Concrete Goals

The seventh and final motivator in OPYOW is the fact that the end goal is very tangible and concrete. That is to say the goal is not abstract, numerical, statistical, digital, etc. Being able to physically pull your own weight is something all kids can see live and in person, hear (the inevitable groans in the last couple of reps), smell (the sweat), and feel (their bodies moving up and down and finally running out of gas). Pull ups require no formula, no interpretation, no pie charts or graphs to explain. Just count 'em out, 1, 2, 3, 4, 5, 6, etc.

Winning the War on Childhood Obesity

These seven motivational factors work together synergistically in order to motivate OPYOW participants to work regularly (twice a week), eat right, get enough rest at night, avoid tobacco, alcohol, and drugs (they make you weak), and finally to take the responsibility for doing these things yourself, because nobody else can do them for you. In short, these seven factors combine to motivate kids to eat better, exercise more, and to naturally immunize themselves against obesity for life. What more can you ask for?

*By the way, these seven motivational pistons can be used to motivate kids to learn reading, writing, and arithmetic as well as the social and emotional skills they need to live strong and fulfilling lives. You can, for example, experiment by substituting "reading" in place of pull ups in this essay and nothing changes. If you set the stage the same way, your kids will be motivated to do the things they need to do to become strong readers. It's all in the way the stage is set.

**Along this same line, the physical experience of learning to do pull ups in small steps, over a period of time serves as a marvelous "Advance Organizer" or mental scaffolding upon which other skills can be efficiently organized, built, learned, and eventually incorporated into a child's tool chest of life. Think of it as a Christmas tree upon which different sets of lights (new knowledge) are organized and understood.

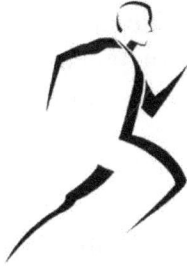

3

What Happens When the Going Gets Tough?

A reader recently wrote in and said, "I understand why you start each participant out at a level where they're guaranteed to succeed. I also understand why you use very small increments of progress/change, and restrict the amount of progress each participant is allowed to make in any one workout. And I understand why you want the leg assisted pull ups to be done in front of the kid's peers and teachers."

"By doing these things you guarantee that all participants will experience a little success every time they workout for many workouts, and many weeks before things get very challenging. You're building in positive expectations, patterns of success experienced in public, boatloads of confidence producing psychological capital, and then you allow the resulting high fives from peers to motivate, inspire, and to help kids learn to look forward to their next opportunity to get on the bar and to get stronger with their friends."

"What I fail to understand is what happens when the easy phase wears off and the whole thing becomes challenging. I mean immunizing themselves against obesity by learning to do pull ups is tough for most kids these days. So I want to know what happens when the going gets tough?"

Excellent Question...

First let me thank to the reader for a great question. Then let me confess, the reader's correct when he says that the easy phase eventually wears off and the whole thing inevitably becomes challenging for most kids. I also understand that as a society, we've become too used to seeing kids giving up when the going gets tough, and refusing to try for fear of humiliating themselves in public. Humiliation after all is un-cool, and all kids want to be cool and accepted by their peers. For most it's their highest priority.

But in years of working with OPYOW I don't ever recall seeing even one child become discouraged and/or refusing to try. And the reasons for that certainly begin with the fact that we intentionally build public success into the experience. More specifically, if the stage is set correctly each child will experience success (grow a little bit stronger) for many consecutive workouts, many consecutive weeks, and often for several months before things get real challenging.

Psychological Capital in the Experiential Bank

But eventually the going gets tough. It's inevitable. And when that happens each child should have weeks and weeks of public success under their belt. By this time the child should have a real good feel for what they're doing, and with an abundance of positive psychological capital stored up in their experiential banks (1) they can grab hold of the bar expecting to succeed just like they've done workout after workout, for weeks and weeks now.

Not only that, but the entire peanut gallery is expecting them to succeed because that's precisely what has happened every time they've touched the bar for a dozen weeks or more. Why should this time be any different?

The Peanut Gallery is Cheering Everyone On

The peanut gallery has also grown used to congratulating each participant when they're done, and they expect to do it again this time. That means they cheer and urge their peers to keep on keeping on, especially when the going gets tough. And when your friends are cheering you on it's really hard to give up, or to quit until you get your chin up to the bar just like everyone expects you to do.

The Psychological Chemistry is Suddenly Reversed

As a matter of fact, under these conditions, with everybody cheering you on, and expecting you to succeed, it's humiliating and it's un-cool to quit without giving it at least 1000%. So you don't quit. You give it 1000%. And when you do the odds of success are increased by approximately the same percentage.

Let me repeat this one more time so you don't miss it. Under these circumstances the psychological chemistry of pull ups is suddenly reversed. It's gone from REFUSING TO TRY for fear of being humiliated in front of your friends, to REFUSING TO GIVE UP for fear of being humiliated in front of your friends. Now how cool is that?

An Increased Challenge Hardens the Resolve

As a matter of fact, in my experiences with OPYOW, when the stage is set right, an increased challenge produces an increase in the child's resolve to succeed. In other words when you're used to succeeding in public, and all your friends are expecting you to succeed in public, odds are that you're going dig down deep enough to find a way to continue succeeding in public.

It's cool to get stronger week after week, month after month. It's cool to be able to tackle a difficult task in front of your friends and succeed. And as the going gets tougher, the success becomes more fulfilling. Not only that but it's fun and you don't want to lose that fun, that cool, or that feeling of being a winner. And when you know the only thing standing between you and the goal line is a little more effort, it's not all that tough for most kids to dig down a little deeper and to come up with a little more.

It's All About Relentless Persistence

And in OPYOW, that's what happens when the going gets tough. We all come together. We all root for one another. And we all carry the ball across the goal line and celebrate each other's win because it's cool to be strong, it's cool to succeed, and it's really fun when we can all be cool, strong, and succeed together. When pull ups finally evolve into a team sport, everyone wins. Oh yes we do.

1. With enough psychological capital stored up in their experiential banks, children can afford to risk hitting a bump in the road without fearing humiliation or embarrassment. As a kid once told me, "If I don't get it this time Coach, I'll get it next time. I promise."

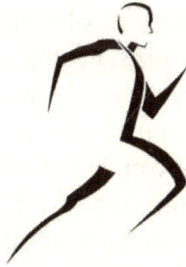

4

Motivational Momentum to Relentless Persistence

As we've said on previous occasions, the three most important factors in any physical fitness routine are motivation, motivation, and motivation. And Operation Pull Your Own Weight (OPYOW) is no exception to that rule.

In other words, if the kids you're working with really want to get a little bit stronger on the pull up bar week after week, month after month the odds of those kids immunizing themselves against obesity for life and winning the war on childhood obesity are enhanced dramatically. On the other hand, if they really don't care, the odds of winning are not worth talking about.

In this sense, OPYOW is all about one thing, motivating kids and keeping them motivated until they're all the way across the finish line. In this light I'd like to introduce you to a concept that some have called motivational momentum. Outside the basic mechanics of learning to how do pull ups, motivational momentum is the single most important concept in the OPYOW lexicon. Motivate kids and everyone wins.

Observing Momentum

Let's begin with a couple of simple observations on the concept of momentum. We've all seen football, basketball, and baseball teams that are on a roll, and every break seems to be going their way. Similarly in Las Vegas gamblers get on a winning streak and they try to ride that streak as long as they can. In politics this animal is simply known as "Big Mo"…when the wind is at your back and things are trending in your favor. And as any politician will readily confess, it's pretty hard to beat Big Mo.

Momentum then is a series of experiences which form a pattern. This pattern in turn translates into expectations, a sense of predictability, even inevitability that's normally absent from the moment. And if you set the stage right, that's precisely what you'll create for kids working on the pull up bar. They'll have an expectation of success that presents itself in the form of confidence and the ability to give 110% in front of their peers, without risking humiliation, and without risking their cool. They'll be on a roll.

Step One – Start Easy

So the first rule of OPYOW is, START EASY. Lower the straps to a level where you know Tommie or Susie will easily be able to do eight (don't let them do nine or ten) leg assisted pull ups (jumping and pulling at the same time) and succeed in front of the class. Call that level their starting point, and when they're finished doing their eight reps, encourage their classmates to celebrate with high fives. The teacher can even pitch in with a pat on the back. In other words when they're done with their leg assisted pull ups workout they should feel successful and proud of themselves.

If you started them off at the right (easy enough) level, each participant will be able to do nine reps in workout # 2, ten reps in workout # 3, eleven reps in workout # 4, and twelve reps in workout # 5.* When they've successfully performed twelve reps at level one, you raise the bar/straps ONE INCH for workout # 6 and start the entire eight to twelve routine all over again. Notice that OPYOW uses very small increments of progress to cultivate success week after week, month after month, which is the experience we call motivational momentum.

It Eventually Becomes Challenging

However, lets' note that this "start 'em easy" formula does not mean that learning to do conventional pull ups is easy from start to finish. Odds are that there will come a point when the task becomes challenging enough that it will require 110% from the young participant. But if that challenge comes along in the wake of 8, 10, or 12 consecutive weeks of success on the bar, and high five's from their friends, these kids will have established a pattern of success, a motivational momentum that will help them to dig in and give it 110%, just like they did last time and the time before.

158

In other words, with motivational momentum in their sails participants tend to give it 110% time after time which increases their odds of success exponentially. And if for some reason they're unable to pop that one more rep this time, the odds of them coming back next time and giving it their all are real good.

Motivational Momentum and Relentless Persistence

Eventually motivational momentum becomes transformed into a phenomenon we like to call relentless persistence. And once armed with the habit of relentless persistence, students will succeed at pull ups, and almost anything else at which they want to succeed. That is to say, cultivate those seeds of motivational momentum for long enough and they'll grow into trees of relentless persistence, tall, straight, and strong. Can an educator do any better by a student? Not in my book he can't

*With two workouts per week on non-consecutive days, five workouts will cover two and a half weeks of success after success after success. And nothing succeeds like success.

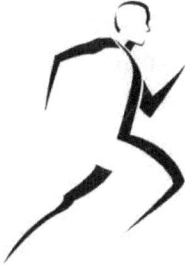

5

Intrinsic VS Extrinsic Motivation

On a number of occasions we've made a point of our preference for "intrinsic" over "extrinsic" motivation in Operation Pull Your Own Weight. However as I write this sentence there is still plenty of confusion between the two in conventional circles. So right from the get go let's recognize that the primary difference is found in who controls the reward. Is it you or is it someone else?

You VS Them...

More specifically if the reason you perform a certain action (say attending school or going to a job) is to gain access to a reward (say good grades or a paycheck) that is controlled by someone other than yourself (say the teacher or the boss) then your action is nothing more than a MEANS to an END outside of the action itself. And under these conditions, whoever controls the end also controls (and can manipulate) the means.

On the other hand, if the reason you perform a certain action (say playing the piano) is because you value the experience itself, you just love doing it, and you actively choose to do it on your own, then the action is intrinsically valued and it cannot be controlled or manipulated by someone other than yourself. In this instance you are intrinsically motivated and your autonomy is not being threatened.

But When Someone Pays You...

But, when someone begins to pay you (reward you) money in order to play the piano (or to do whatever you value intrinsically) there's the danger of your intrinsic motivation being undermined. That is to say, if your focus changes from the sheer joy of playing the piano to the money that can be generated as the result of playing the piano, then whoever controls the money can manipulate and control your piano playing. At this point your intrinsic motivation (your independence and autonomy) has been undermined/ sacrificed to the extrinsic reward.

How Does This Apply to OPYOW?

So you might ask, how does all this apply to Operation Pull Your Own Weight? The answer is that if a child is motivated by their natural desire to become stronger and more independent and they actively choose to do pull ups in order to accommodate that desire, they are intrinsically motivated and they are not being manipulated or controlled by some alien force outside of themselves. They are acting autonomously.

But If Dad Pays Johnny...

On the other hand if Dad starts paying Johnny a quarter for every pull up he performs, there's the danger of Johnny becoming focused on the money as opposed to the experience of growing stronger week after week, month after month. And if that happens then Johnny is no longer in the driver's seat. Dad is suddenly in control and he can manipulate Johnny and his pull ups by manipulating the reward. He can even eliminate the reward altogether at which point Johnny's extrinsic motivation to continue doing pull ups will be eliminated and the action itself will be extinguished. Under these conditions is it any wonder why OPYOW favors intrinsic motivation over extrinsic motivation?

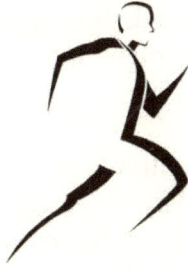

6

The Habit of Winning!

Winning can become a habit if you're willing to start right now, (the earlier the better) and redefine winning as "Becoming a little stronger today than you were yesterday, a little stronger this week than you were last week, a little stronger this month than last month, and a lot stronger this year than last year." While you're at it, redefine losing as "Failing to become stronger day after day, week after week, month after month, and year after year."

Becoming the Captain of Your Own Ship

Under these conditions nobody else controls your opportunities to become a winner or a loser. The cards are all in your hands, and not in the hands of a conventional competitor, a teacher, a coach, a boss, a manager, a drill sergeant, or any other authority figure.

You become your own authority figure. You determine whether you'll develop the habit of winning or the habit of losing. That is to say, nobody can prevent you from becoming habitually stronger. In fact the mere act of taking personal control of your own ship is the second and arguably the most important step in developing the habit of winning.

Fulfilling Your Own Potential

Think about this one. Show me a kid who starts young (say kindergarten) and spends twelve consecutive years cultivating the habit of winning, day after day, week after week, month after month, until he or she graduates from high school, and I'll show you a graduate who has come frighteningly close to fulfilling his or her

163

potential – a winning ideal that today's educational institutions only dream about. On the other hand, this ideal is immediately accessible to any child who focuses their attention on self competition.

On the Contrary

On the contrary, by actively pitting kids against each other starting at a very early age (say kindergarten) the current system does a great job of creating a handful of winners at the top of the educational ladder, a bunch of also-rans (average students) in the middle, and another handful of losers struggling to hang on to the bottom rung of the ladder.

Realistically by virtue of defining winning and losing in conventional terms this hierarchical conclusion is mathematically inevitable. It's the only possible result. Then we sit around and wonder how the USA has managed to become a society in which a small percentage of the population can wield almost infinite power, while everyone else struggles. The answer is - this result is systematically built into our institutions, starting with the institution of education.

Redefining Winning

On the other hand, there's also nothing to stop educational institutions from redefining winning and losing in a way that encourages every single student to develop his or her full potential every day, every week, every month, all year long. And if helping develop the potential of every single student to the max is not education's main goal, there's something dramatically wrong with the system we refer to as "education."

Winning, Losing, and Childhood Obesity Prevention

Now, how does the habit of winning or losing impact the issue of childhood obesity prevention? Well, for starters, show me a kid who's successfully cultivated the habit of winning and I'll show you a kid who does not suffer from self esteem issues – the exact problem upon which so much of childhood obesity feeds and grows.

A kid who's developed the habit of winning has also developed the psychological strength to say "no" to things that undermine his or her well being whether tobacco, alcohol, drugs, or fat filled fast food. They can say "no" with conviction and make it stick because they've made self control, self determination, and winning a lifelong habit. It's seeped into the DNA over time and the results are tangible and measurable.

In other words, these kids are in the habit of saying "yes" to those things that make them strong. They're in the habit of saying yes to winning. And as the old saying goes, "Everybody loves a winner." So why not choose winning over losing, especially since it's well within your power to do exactly that?

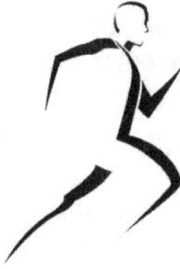

7

Frequent Progress Equals Big Motivation

If you go on a diet and lose a pound a day your motivation to continue will be sky high. If your weight loss drops off to a pound a week, your motivation takes a serious hit. And if it drops off to a pound a month, it's all but out the door, right?

If you're an investor and the stocks you choose yield daily gains your motivation to continue investing will be sky high. If your gains drop off to once a week, your motivation takes a serious hit. And if your gains dwindle down to once a month or once a year you'll probably be looking for some different stocks to invest in.

If you're a professional baseball player who gets a hit every other time you make a trip to the plate, you're motivation to get back in the batter's box will be sky high. If that frequency is reduced to once every fourth trip to the plate your motivation takes a serious hit. But if the frequency drops down to one hit for every ten trips to the plate, you'll be considering retirement in the near future.

The Moral of These Three Scenarios

The moral of these three scenarios is simply that motivation is heavily dependent on the frequency of progress in whatever it is you're looking to achieve. In fact they're related in such a way that when one side of the ledger goes up, the other one does the same. When one side goes down, the other follows suit. This is true enough that the entire concept of motivation can be boiled down to a formula that reads Frequent Progress (FP) = Big Motivation (BM).

How, you might ask, does this formula fit into the field of childhood obesity prevention? For starters the concept of progress implies measurement of some kind. And in the field of childhood obesity there are four conventional tools with which you can measure progress. The first, and most popular (because it's dramatically cheaper that the others) is known as BMI or Body Mass Index, which is a modern 21st century edition of the age old height/weight charts that were used back in the 40's and 50's.

BMI, Skin Fold, Impedance, & Underwater Weighing

Despite the fact that BMI calculations could easily be done more often in childhood obesity programs, you seldom see calculations done more than once a quarter or even once a semester. So the infrequency of feedback, together with the abstract nature of the feedback itself (a cold, hard number) means that using BMI as the measurement tool in any childhood obesity program offers almost NO MOTIVATIONAL VALUE whatsoever for participating kids. And voids in motivation automatically produce failure.

Two other conventional measurement tools that are used much less frequently than BMI include the skin fold method, and electronic impedance. Even when they are used (for a variety of reasons), you seldom see them used more frequently than BMI. So once again, the lack of meaningful frequency means that the skin fold method, and electronic impedance also offer NO MOTIVATIONAL VALUE whatsoever to kids.

The final conventional option is known as underwater weighing, and its greatest benefit is that, when done correctly, it's significantly more accurate than any of the other three conventional options. But due to its labor intensity and expense, underwater weighing is seldom found outside the university physiology lab. Due to the infrequency of its use, underwater weighing is unworthy of consideration when it comes to motivation.

Function, the Unconventional Measuring Tool

The fifth, and most unconventional measurement tool one has at his/her disposal is function. That is to say, how high can you jump? How fast can you run? How far can you run? How may pull ups can you do? How many dips can you do? How many hand stand push ups can you do? More specifically, changes (improvements or deteriorations) in functional ability directly reflect changes in physical efficiency/body composition.

For a variety of reasons, at Operation Pull Your Own Weight we've chosen to use pull ups (dips work just as well) as the activity

168

with which we measure changes in physical efficiency/body composition. Our contention is that pull ups automatically reward fat loss with performance gain, and they automatically punishes fat gain with performance loss. Conversely, performance increases automatically reflect percentage of fat losses, and performance losses automatically reflect percentage of fat increases.

Start Easy and Use Small Increments of Progress

And if the stage is set correctly, kid's frequency of progress will be extremely high along with the motivation levels that accompany success. The whole idea is to find a starting point at which success in front of their peers is certain, and to limit progress to very small increments in order to insure that progress is made every time a child grabs the pull up bar (I'm stronger) week after week, month after month, all year long. The whole idea is to create a pattern in which kids learn to expect success instead of failure.

On the basis of motivation alone, measuring functional performance instead of meaningless, abstract entities like BMI or percentage of body fat (kids don't understand it and they don't care about it) offers humongous advantages over all four conventional methods. And by the way, it's all about motivation. If you lose the motivational war, your odds of winning the childhood obesity prevention war are slimmer than slim.

Just Remember FP = BM

Just remember, FP = BM or Frequency of Progress equals Big Motivation. Cover the motivational base and you're well on your way to accomplishing some big things on behalf of the kids that you work with.

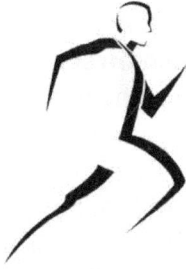

8

Choosing to Lose

I've stated on many occasions that we don't have losers in Operation Pull Your Own Weight. But I'd like to clarify that statement by saying this doesn't mean the possibility of losing does not exist. Instead it means, of all the kids I've ever seen participate in OPYOW, I've yet to actually see a loser.

In this light, OPYOW defines winning as growing a little stronger this week than you were last week, a little stronger this month than last month, and a lot stronger this year than last year. In other words, if you fail to grow stronger this week, this month, and this year, you have lost an opportunity to grow stronger. And in the event this scenario actually occurs, you would be considered a loser in OPYOW.

The Only Way to Lose is...

But the only way you fail to get a little stronger week after week, month after month is by failing to apply yourself, failing to try. When you fail to try, then failing (losing) becomes the automatic default, the self-fulfilling prophecy. That is to say in the real world nobody improves or wins without trying.

Now, think about this. Under these conditions the strongest, fastest, and most athletically gifted kid in town becomes a loser if he fails to try and he fails to fulfill his potential. On the other hand, the weakest, slowest, and most un-athletic kid in town easily becomes a winner by applying himself and by making a little progress every week, every month, all year long. In this context then, winning and losing become functions of one's own choosing, one's ability to take responsibility for oneself.

Everyone Has it Within His Power

Under these conditions the naturally gifted athlete can easily deteriorate and become a non athlete, while the non-athlete can systematically choose to grow stronger, faster, and more athletic. In the long run the non-athlete who applies himself becomes a winner at the expense of the athlete who inadvertently chooses to lose. That's how anyone can lose in OPYOW. That's also how anyone can win in OPYOW.

To quote Louis L'Amour from his classic The Walking Drum, "Everyone has it within his power to say this I am today, and that I shall be tomorrow." We all have it within our reach to fulfill our potentials and to become winners in the process. Why would anyone actually choose to lose?

*This systematic, built in losing is more the rule than the exception in our nation's schools today.

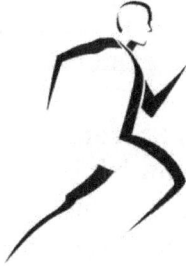

9

Strong at Everything, Weak at Nothing

I confess, I want to be strong (i.e. independent, self-reliant, resilient) at everything and weak at nothing. And furthermore I confess that I've never met another human being who wants to be weak at anything. In other words, every person I've ever known wants to be strong (1) at everything and weak at nothing. There are no exceptions to this rule.

Physically Strong

In my vocabulary, strong is always good, while weak is always bad, regardless of what you're talking about. For example, I want to be physically strong in order to run fast and far, jump high (tall buildings in a single bound), move quickly from side to side, climb tall mountains, and to rescue damsels in distress.

Mentally Strong

I also want to be strong (2) mentally. I want to be able to read great literature whether it's the Bible, the Koran, Shakespeare, Milton, Melville, Whitman, Twain, or Faulkner and understand everything I read. I also want to be able to handle numbers like a human computer. And I want to be able to express myself clearly, concisely, insightfully, and in Technicolor when and if the occasion calls for it. Yes, mental strength is a great virtue in my book.
Spiritually, Socially, Emotionally, and Psychologically Strong

I also want to be spiritually, socially, emotionally, and psychologically strong. And there's absolutely nothing at which I want to be weak. In this sense I, like all humans want to be Superman, Uberman, or God, who is by definition the alpha and the

173

omega, the top and the bottom, the essence of essences, and obviously strong at everything and weak at nothing.

Exponentially Stronger and Stronger

But alas, no matter how hard I work, or how strong I become in how many different ways, as an individual human being my strength has limitations. I'm not Superman, Uberman, or God, and I never expect to be. On the other hand I've also discovered that when I help someone else become stronger, I can actually feel my own strength increasing.

In fact when one person is helping another become stronger over time, that relationship is generally considered to be unique. In my experience, most people don't have many of these kinds of relationships in their lives. And when they do have one it stands out as something special and it's valued highly by both parties. It's the essence of a genuine parent-child, teacher-pupil, or coach-player relationship, and the only reason some people stay in the education field at all.

Furthermore, when I help a number of others become stronger, I find that my own strength increases even more significantly. And when those others go out and help others become stronger, my strength increases exponentially. In the midst of such a multi-level pursuit of strength, the very idea of growing stronger becomes contagious, it rubs off on others, and it spreads like a virus, a spark in a bone dry forest.

From Contagious to Radioactive

When enough people are helping enough other people grow stronger in a variety of ways, the entire atmosphere becomes super charged, super contagious, and it evolves into another stage that I like to describe as "Radioactive." Yes, when a group moves beyond contagiousness and into Redioactiveness, you'll see a tipping point, a movement (i.e. civil rights, feminism), a miracle. And in the midst of this kind of miraculous experience you'll come frighteningly close to knowing yourself in the most fully human sense.

1. The Relativity of Strength

In this essay we're using the term strength in a relative sense. That is to say, someone who carries a heavy load needs a lot more

174

strength than someone who carries a light load. For example, there are two people capable of doing 10 pull ups. One of them weighs 200 lbs and the other weighs only 100 lbs. Regardless of the fact that the 200 pound fellow needs twice as much brute strength to perform the same 10 pull ups, their relative strength is exactly the same. And if the bigger guy loses 50 pounds of excess weight, his performance and his relative strength will increase significantly even though his brute strength remains unchanged. Relative strength is all about what you can do.

2. The Purpose of Strength

The purpose of strength in this essay is to underwrite and insure freedom, independence, self reliance, integrity, and dignity of the individual. Furthermore it serves to avoid him/her ever becoming a burden on others, and to maximize his/her odds of being able to help others grow stronger week after week, month after month, year after year. More specifically it aims to discourage and to undermine privilege or hierarchy of any kind. This is the kind of mutually respectful strength that a democracy is built on.

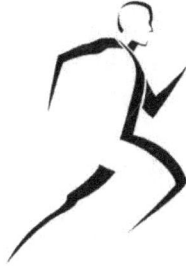

10

Enlightened Self Interest

In one sense, the philosophical centerpiece of a childhood obesity prevention strategy is a concept known as "Enlightened Self Interest." This concept suggests that adults have a moral obligation to become as strong as they can, in as many ways as they can, in order to become as self sufficient as they can, and to minimize the odds of becoming dependent on others. More specifically, full fledged adults are obligated to give this self sufficiency goal no less than a 100% effort. And if they give less than 100%, they have no business expecting others to lend them a helping hand when they occasionally stumble and fall.

Keeping Your Feet on Solid Ground

Inherent in the concept of enlightened self interest is the recognition that taking responsibility for oneself imparts a sense of dignity and self-respect on the individual who's taking that responsibility. And it's also fully understood that this dignity and self respect is one form of compensation, a great motivator that can't be expressed in dollars and cents by some corporate accountant on Wall Street or on Main Street. It's simply not for sale at any price, it can't be given as a gift, so the only way you can get it is to earn it. That makes it a very important form of compensation.

Also inherent in the concept of enlightened self interest is the recognition that when someone is scrambling to take care of their own affairs, it's difficult if not impossible to help anyone else take care of theirs. In other words, if you know someone who's drowning and you want to throw them a lifeline, you'd better have both feet planted solidly on dry land, or be one really strong swimmer. But if you're in the water yourself, flailing away for your own life, the odds of you helping anyone else in any way are negligible at best.

In the context of enlightened self interest, strong is always good, and weak is always bad. Helping someone else get stronger then is the height of virtue, a privilege, a payoff, and an ROI all at the same time.

Encourages Efficiency and Discourages Excess

Enlightened self interest also recognizes that strength is a relative concept. For example, it takes twice as much upper body pulling strength for a 200 pound athlete to do 5 pull ups as it does for a 100 pound athlete to do 5 pull ups. As a matter of fact the relative upper body pulling strength of a 100 pound athlete who can do 10 pull ups is DOUBLE the relative strength of a 200 pound athlete who can only do 5 pull ups. Enlightened self interest thus applauds efficiency and discourages excess of almost any kind.

For example, from both an economic and an environmental perspective, enlightened self interest was well represented by Native American Indians who were well known for the "understanding" they had with Mother Nature. It said something like, "If we avoid taking more buffalo than we need, you will continue to provide us with an abundance of buffalo." In this context nature and greed are inevitably mortal enemies. When we systematically encourage greed and arrogance there will eventually be a high price to pay.

Flip Sides of the Same Coin

From a linguistic perspective, enlightened self interest recognizes that in order to explain, define, and to understand individuality, concepts like family, group, team, and collective are necessary. After all, what is an individual if not the opposite of a group or a team? On the other hand what is a group or a team if not a collection of individuals?

Much like the heads and tails on a quarter flipped to start a football game, individuality and collectivity are opposite sides of the same coin. To talk in terms of the importance of one without recognizing the importance of the other is overlooking the blatantly obvious.

Enlightened VS Plain Old Self Interest

At bottom, there's a humongous difference between enlightened self interest, and the plain old garden variety "me first and to hell with you" self interest, also known as selfishness, self centeredness, self righteousness, and arrogance. These are all forms of shortsightedness, if not moral ignorance and stupidity.

We're All in This Together

In contrast, enlightened self interest understands and identifies with those who say things like "What's good for my family is good for me. What's good for my neighborhood is good for my family. What's good for my city is good for my neighborhood. What's good for my county, state, nation, world, is good for my neighborhood." Arrogance lacks that kind of understanding.

Those who operate from the perspective of enlightened self interest also understand when someone says, "We're all in this together, so if I can help my kids get strong, that's good for me. If I can help my neighborhood get strong, that's good for my spouse and kids. If I can help my city get strong, that's good for my neighborhood, etc."

Hats off to Strong Kids

So we contend that it's critically important to recognize that ALL KIDS want to be strong at everything and weak at nothing, and that it's the obligation of adults who work with kids (parents, teachers, etc.) to cultivate that desire, and to help all kids come as close to fulfilling their natural born strengths/potentials as possible.

Thus individual strength is the basic building block for enlightened self interest. Without a foundation of strength and confidence, the odds of kids evolving beyond a natural and immature self centeredness to the level of enlightened self interest are bleak. Therefore, let's all salute and applaud anything and everything that produces STRONG KIDS!

Section 6

Logistical Issues Addressed

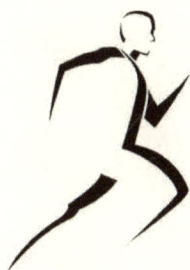

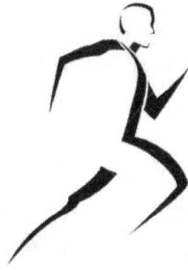

1

Childhood Obesity as a Strategic Priority in Schools

In a school system, how do you know what's really important? The answer to this question is, you take a look at their website, check out their mission statements, and see what they've recognized as strategic priorities for the school year. This will tell you in black and white what's really important to this school system, and what's less important.

When the administrative cadre, including school principals administrate, they do so with those strategic priorities in mind. In other words, once those items are set in stone for the school year, everything else becomes secondary and of lesser importance to the principal, and in turn to the teachers, the teaching assistants, and to the students.

Do a Quick Google Search

In this light we can now consider the fate of the childhood obesity epidemic in the hands of school systems across the USA. Try this for starters. Do a quick Google search for school system websites in your local area. When you get there drill down until you find their mission statement, and their list of strategic goals and priorities and see how many of them have mentioned anything at all about childhood obesity.

It Won't Buy a Cup of Coffee

My bet is that you could include the entire nation in this search and if you were given a dime for every one you found that mentioned childhood obesity at all, it would hardly be enough to buy a cup of coffee at McDonalds. In other words, if childhood obesity is almost never recognized as a strategic goal or priority by local school boards or their administrative brass, then it's annually placed on the back burner and it continually fails to get the attention required to turn the tide and begin to win the war.

The Stakes are Already Incredibly High

This is the case despite the fact that obesity and related problems cost our nation $215 billion annually according to the latest Brookings Institute figures. This is the case despite the fact that this epidemic is exponentially bigger than all previous epidemics combined. The Pentagon has labeled it a national security threat. And in the case of schools themselves obesity has been proven to undermine academic achievement, encourage anti-social behaviors like taunting and bullying, which in turn impacts attendance – the very basis for school funding.

So What Will it Take???

If all this fails to grab the undivided attention of school boards and administrators, the question becomes, what will it take to finally make childhood obesity a strategic priority in our nation's schools? What will it take to light a fire under educational leaders and for them to give a green light to physical educators (and others) to take action against what the US Center for disease control has called "Our nation's number one health threat?" In the words of Mahatma Ghandi, "Action exposes priorities."

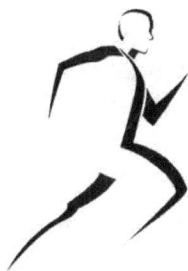

2

Resolving the Problem of Limited Time

We've had a number of Physical Educators tell us they'd like to start an Operation Pull Your Own Weight childhood obesity prevention program, but they've each had a plateful of existing mandates – one of which was not childhood obesity prevention – and a limited amount of time in which to cover their existing bases.

Under these conditions the question became, how do you fit an additional new activity like OPYOW into a curriculum that's already bulging at the seams? The creative, big picture answer was, "Where there's a will there's a way."

Three Stations Generate Expediency

In a brainstorming session, one suggested they each install a ten foot long, wall mounted pull up bar in each of their respective gyms. Then on each ten foot bar they'd mount three sets of height adjustable pull up straps, which would give them three stations on which three students could perform leg assisted pull ups simultaneously.

Color Coded Higher and Higher

Next, for the sake of expediency, they decided to dispense with the daily documentation that's normally required in OPYOW. In lieu of the daily documentation they color coded and positioned each set of height adjustable straps so that there were 6" differentials between them. The RED set, for example, was positioned low enough that everyone could easily do at least 8 leg assisted pull ups. The BLUE set was positioned 6" higher, while the YELLOW set was positioned 6" higher yet.*

With this new equipment in place, they could work leg assisted pull ups into their regular warm up routines at the start of each class. They instructed all students to choose and use any set of grips, as long as they could do at least 8 reps. So along with push ups, sit ups, and jumping jacks for example, their students would also do at least 8 leg assisted pull ups (more if possible) right at the start of each and every class.

Progress Automatically Built In

Now here's how they squeezed documented progress into their new strategy. They decided that if they raised each set of grips one inch every other week (two inches each month) the change would go relatively unnoticed by their students. Yet over the course of a school year (nine months) the grips will have been raised a full 18 inches.

The net result would be that even though all students had an easy place to get on board at the beginning, they'd gradually have less and less leg assistance, which makes the exercise itself gradually more and more challenging.

At Year's End

At the end of the current school year they plan to conduct a fitness assessment that will include conventional pull ups. This will allow them to determine what percentage of their students are naturally immunized against obesity for life by virtue of being able to do at least one conventional pull up, and maintaining that ability by eating and exercising in ways that allow them to continue (a functional acid test that can be performed once a week in less than a minute) for a lifetime.

They speculate that, as the result of following this procedure, the percentage of students who are naturally immunized against obesity for life will increase significantly year after year until they've effectively eliminated obesity in their respective schools. We plan to check back in with them at the end of year one.

*These levels obviously have to be adjusted for each grade level. In other words the first grade settings are a little higher than the kindergarten settings. And the second grade settings were a little higher than the first grade settings, etc. Also notice that there's a 12" differential between the highest and the lowest set of grips, with the third in the middle.

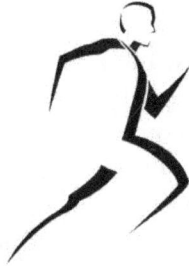

3.

In Less Than Two Minutes Each Week...

In all schools these days, curriculum are bulging at the seams, expectations are running high, class sizes a growing larger, while salaries have stalled in the midst of a stagnant economy. Now someone wants you to seriously consider adding childhood obesity prevention to your already overloaded plate, and no matter how simple, it still feels like the proverbial straw that could break the camel's back.

Two Minutes Per Week...

Now before you hit the eject button let me interject that this little intervention takes less than TWO MINUTES PER WEEK out of each of your student's jam packed schedules. That is to say, out of the 30 plus hours (1800 plus minutes) that students spend in school every week, this activity requires less than TWO MINUTES!

As the result of this weekly two minutes of time and effort you can help your school's students naturally immunize themselves against obesity (and the myriad of related problems including poor academic performance and anti-social behaviors) for life.

You'll Even Increase Test Scores

In other words, if you can figure out where in your curriculum to squeeze TWO MINUTES PER WEEK for each one of your students, you could guarantee that they'll never have to wrestle with America's # 1 health threat, and they'll never have to experience the myriad of social problems (i.e. bullying) that go hand in hand with obesity. On top of that, since obesity has been shown to severely undermine academic performance, you'll also increase the odds of their test scores going up in the process.

To Cash in on This Predictable Dividend

So to cash in on this predictable dividend sitting right out on the horizon, the question becomes, where in your piled high curriculum does this two minute per week activity best fit, most logically fit, most seamlessly fit? Is it in the PE curriculum? Is it in the home room setting? Is it before or after school?

Making the World a Better Place

The answer in school A may be different than in school B or in school C. But surely in the over 1800 minutes you have students each and every week there's a place in which to squeeze these two magical minutes worth of activity. Answer this question and you're in the process of making the quality of life better for your students, their families, your teachers, and the community at large.

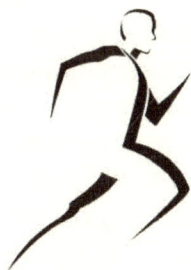

4

Longfellow Elementary Documents Improvements

According to the official Operation Pull Your Own Weight prescription, kids should have access to height adjustable pull up straps twice, or maximally three times a week, on non- consecutive days. Barb Williams, PE Instructor at Longfellow Elementary School in Wheaton gave her 4th and 5th grade students access twice a week.

According to the prescription, the height of the grips and the repetitions should be customized to fit each student, and tightly controlled by the teacher in order to insure weekly progress over many weeks. Weekly progress in turn encourages the motivational momentum upon which OPYOW is built. Williams however allowed her troops to do as many repetitions as they wanted to do, as often as they wanted to do them.

According to the prescription each student's workout should be documented in order to generate an evidence based paper trail and to cost justify this functional, obesity prevention intervention. But at Longfellow Elementary classes are short on time and long on all the bases to be covered. In other words, there was no time for the detailed documentation suggested by the OPYOW prescription.

Growing Stronger is Always Cool
On the other hand, Williams knew intuitively that kids value the opportunity to grow stronger in front of their peers. She also knew that height adjustable straps in conjunction with leg assisted pull ups (jumping and pulling at the same time) give all students the opportunity to succeed, without the humiliation that often goes hand in hand with the inability to do conventional pull ups.

191

The Kids Loved Using Them

At Longfellow leg assisted pull ups were strictly voluntary. No one was forced to participate. "The main thing," according to Williams, "was that the kids just loved using the height adjustable straps (similar to gymnastic rings). And in the process of using them, they developed the upper body pulling strength that so many kids lack these days."

What Williams did document however was her students' BMI scores. She also documented their ability to do conventional pull ups, as well as the percentage of students who won Presidential Fitness Awards. The results are as follows.

Zero Percent Were Obese...

At the end of the school year a whopping 52 percent (78 out of 149) of her 4th and 5th grade students were able to do at least one conventional pull up, and according to their BMI scores NONE of these students were obese. Furthermore, as long as they eat and exercise in ways that allow them to maintain the ability, none will ever have to wrestle with the disability that the US Surgeon General calls "America's # 1 health threat."

Presidential Fitness Awards Up by 60%

Not only that but the percentage of students who won Presidential Fitness Awards increased by 60 percent. "We generally have 30 to 35 winners. But this year we had 54," said Williams. "And it had lots to do with the fact that this year we had more kids who could do pull ups."

Despite their lack of regimentation, Operation Pull Your Own Weight was a success at Longfellow Elementary School this past school year. Not only that, but "OPYOW will be a big part of our curriculum next year," Williams added. Hats off to Barb Williams and her students for taking documented bites out of childhood obesity!

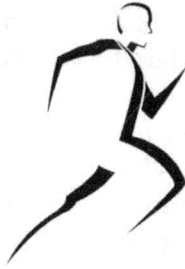

5

Success In the YMCA Setting

If you went on a diet and lost a pound a day, would you consider it a success? Would you be highly motivated to stick with your diet until you reached your ideal body weight? My bet is that you're answering yes, yes, a thousand times yes!!!

Frequent progress is inevitably a strong motivator, whether you're a dieter, a stock market investor who's trying to generate regular, predictable dividends, or kids in Tri-Town YMCA's Operation Pull Your Own Weight program who are learning to do conventional pull ups and in the process to naturally immunize themselves against obesity for life. Simply stated the formula is "Frequent Progress = Big Motivation."

In this light, Chuck Pickerill, Program Director for Tri Town YMCA oversees Operation Pull Your Own Weight, a uniquely practical childhood obesity prevention intervention that began as part of their after school curriculum in February of 2010. The most recent edition began last September, and includes 33 kids (20 boys and13 girls) at Manor Hill and Pleasant Lane Elementary Schools in Lombard.

Documented Progress Generates Motivation

In Pickerill's words, "When we started the program we planned to generate weekly progress with each student. What we've witnessed however is twice our projected progress. The kids workout twice a week and every one of them has made a little progress (by adding another rep, or raising the straps another inch) every single time they've worked out. When kids tackle a difficult task like pull ups and succeed week after week in front of their friends, the motivation just builds exponentially. Needless to say we have no shortage when it comes to learning to do pull ups."

Pull Ups and Obesity Prevention?

Now you may be wondering what exactly do pull ups have to do with childhood obesity prevention? The answer is nothing, except for the statistics confirming that for kids who can perform at least one conventional pull up, the odds of being obese are between zero and zilch. That is to say, you can't have 30% body fat or a 30 BMI score and still do a pull up.

"So if kids can develop the ability to do at least one pull up and maintain it – through good eating and exercise habits – they've naturally immunized themselves against obesity for life," said Pickerill. And that's a pretty big achievement in our view."

So what else can we say about the kids participating in Tri Town Y's OPYOW program? For starters it was originated and financed under the auspices of a local not for profit group known as Healthy Lombard, a village-wide initiative focused on eliminating childhood obesity, promoting healthy living, which hopes to expand its presence in a variety of other DuPage County venues. "We're ecstatic over Tri-Town's success with OPYOW" said Healthy Lombard Founder Jay Wojcik. "Every child in DuPage County should have access to this simple, obesity preventing experience."

Additional Data

Furthermore, 19 out of 33 participants have logged over 20 workouts with the highest being four students in the 25 and 26 workout range. 14 of the 33 participants have raised the bar four inches, 6 have raised it five inches, and two have raised it 6 inches.* "For most kids this age," Pickerill said, "when they've raised the bar 12 inches they're out of leg assistance and they'll be doing conventional pull ups. At the pace these kids are improving we expect about half will be able to do at least one conventional pull up by the end of the school year. And the other half will be well on their way."

"Once they've arrived they'll also be naturally immunized against obesity for life as long as they eat and exercise in ways that allow them to maintain the ability. So, if you want your kids naturally immunized against obesity for life," he said, "make sure they can physically pull their own weight. It's just that simple."

Four Students to be Honored

Four Tri-Town OPYOW students will be honored for their efforts at the Healthy Lombard Fitness February celebration on February 3rd. "This is proof," said Wojcik "that OPYOW is making a legitimate difference. OPYOW really does walk the walk rather than just talk the talk," she added.

*On the average it takes most kids approximately 60 workouts to complete the process, which is effectively about one school year's worth of workouts.

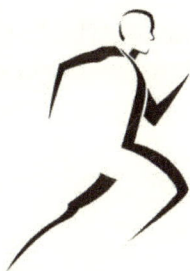

6

Strongville, IA School District Plans to Raise $100,000 by Defeating Childhood Obesity

The Strongville plan has 10 private sector sponsors who will contribute ONE DOLLAR apiece for each student who's naturally immunized against obesity for life.

In other words, they plan to generate $10 for each student who can perform at least one conventional pull up because statistics prove that the odds of kids who can physically pull their own weight being obese are microscopically small. And if they maintain the ability, they've naturally immunized themselves against obesity for life. Check it out.

Year One They Plan to...
1. Make conventional pull ups a part of their existing fitness testing protocol.
2. Identify all those students who can do at least one conventional pull up.
3. Generate $10 (10 X $1 = $10) for each student who can do at least one pull up.
4. Over the school year encourage all those who can do pull ups to maintain the ability.
5. For all those currently unable, they'll help them learn to do at least one pull up.

Year Two They Plan to...
1. Make conventional pull ups a part of their existing fitness testing protocol.

2. Identify all those new students who have developed the ability to do at least one pull up since last year and <u>generate an additional $10 for each new member</u>.

3. Over the school year encourage all those who can do pull ups to maintain the ability.

4. For all those who are currently unable, help them learn to do at least one pull up.

Years Three and Four They Plan to...
1. Repeat year two's strategy until childhood obesity is eliminated completely in Strongville School District. Then they'll celebrate their achievements.

FOR EXAMPLE, for the sake of round numbers say the district has 10,000 students, and 25% (2500) can do at least one pull up - they'll generate $25,000 in the first year.

If they double that percentage in year two, (from 25% to 50%) they'll generate an additional $25,000

In year three if they're up to 75%, they'll generate an additional $25,000.

In year four if they're up to 100%, they'll generate an additional $25,000.

$100,000 in Four Years by Beating Childhood Obesity...
So, presuming Strongville School District has 10,000 students, they'll generate $100,000 in four years, and eliminate the childhood obesity epidemic in the process. Can anyone even imagine a more impressive return on any investment?

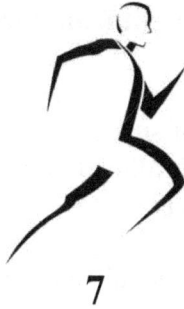

Strongville Fund Raiser FAQ's

Q. So why would anyone wait around hoping and praying for a grant to finally materialize when they can EASILY raise the funds they need by PROACTIVELY BEATING CHILDHOOD OBESITY along with all kinds of related problems?

A. We have no good answer to that question.

Q. What do pull ups have to do with beating childhood obesity?

A. Statistics prove that the odds of kids who can physically pull their own weight (do at least one conventional pull up) being obese are microscopically small. Furthermore, given access to the right info and experiences, most kids can be inspired to develop the ability to do pull ups in one school year or less. And if they maintain the ability (which requires decent eating and exercise habits) they will have naturally immunized themselves against obesity for life.

Q. What are the sponsors' obligations? What are they expected to do?

A. Sponsors are responsible for contributing/pledging ONE DOLLAR for each student who naturally immunizes themselves against obesity by learning to physically pull their own weight (do at least one conventional pull up.) The maximum contribution/pledge for any one sponsor is $2,500 annually for four consecutive school years.

Q. How does a sponsor benefit from their participation? What's their motivation?

A. They'll be recognized for supporting a local school system that can prove they're beating childhood obesity. Can you imagine a better community based ROI?

Q. Who's responsible for recruiting the private sector sponsor?

A. Although it's an excellent project for a local PTA that's interested in raising funds and beating childhood obesity all at the same time, for the first 10 participating school systems the Pull Your Own Weight Foundation will cover that base. The organizers will earn a percentage of the proceeds in return for the time and effort they spend organizing this event.

Q. What do I (as a Physical Educator) have to do in order to raise these funds?

A. You simply add pull ups to your existing annual fitness testing protocol, collect the data on the enclosed sheets (or print it out on your own spreadsheets if that's easier), and give your results to the PYOW Foundation. **NOTHING ELSE IS REQUIRED OF YOU.**

Q. Which grip should I have my kids use?

A. Use any grip. For the purposes of this project Pull Ups and Chin Ups are synonymous. Just make sure they start from all the way down (elbows straight) and then pull all the way up (chin touching the bar). That covers all the bases as far as we're concerned.

Appendix

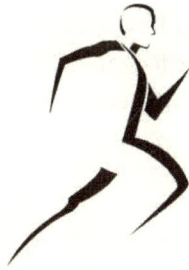

1

Functional Obesity Risk Evaluation/FORE Score

Equipment Required:
• One pull up bar
• One set of height adjustable suspension training straps (see page 99 of this book)
• A wall mounted tape measure that extends approximately eight feet high.

Step 1: Using the tape, measure and record the level (the inch) where the participant's CHIN touches the tape. That will be the low point so let's designate that point L.

Step 2: Ask the participant to reach into the air as high as possible, measure and record the level (the inch) at which their FINGER TIPS touch the tape. That will be the high point so let's designate that point H.

Step 3: Lower the height adjustable straps/grips down to a level where the participant can EASILY do ONE LEG ASSISTED PULL UP (jumping and pulling at the same time/see page 99 of this book) and hold it for a one count before letting themselves back down to the ground. Presuming that was very easy, gradually raise the grips in small increments, while asking the participant to do one more leg assisted pull up at each stop. Eventually this becomes challenging. When you find a level where the participant can still do one good leg assisted pull up but can go no higher, refer to the tape measure and record the level (the inch) where the grips touch the tape. That will be the middle point so let's designate that point M.

Step 4: Now, perform the following calculations.
• Subtract L from H in order to get X (H – L = X)
• Subtract L from M in order to get Y (M - L = Y)
• Divide X into Y in order to get an individual's FORE Score (X/Y = FORE Score)

Example # 1

Presuming participant # 1 is unable to do any conventional pull ups, calculate the difference between their H and L which gives you X. Let's say X is 24 inches.

Next, calculate the difference between their M and L which gives you Y. Let's say that Y is 12 inches.

With these two figures in hand, divide the participant's Y by their X (12/24) and you'll find their FORE Score is 50%. That means participant # 1 is half way to being able to perform conventional pull ups - at which point they're naturally immunized against obesity. (If the difference was 18" instead of 12" their FORE is 75%. If it was 6" the FORE is 25%, etc.).

Example # 2

In the process of completing Step 3, you'll occasionally find participants who are strong and light enough to perform at least one conventional, unassisted pull up. When this occurs their FORE Score is 100%. Five pull ups = 500%. Ten pull ups = 1000%, etc. And with a FORE Score more is always better.

The Relationship Between BMI and FORE

At this point the question becomes, why use two measurements instead of just one? The answer is that BMI and FORE have different strengths that actually compliment one another. BMI's greatest strengths include the fact that it's a universally accepted, non-invasive metric, and it's inexpensive/cost effective on the front end.

On the other hand, a FORE Score's greatest strength is that it accurately reflects changes in body fat and muscle mass – which BMI does not. FORE is equally non-invasive and inexpensive/cost effective on the front AND THE BACK END.

Why Combine BMI and FORE?

The virtue of combining these two metrics is that if/when a participant's FORE Score reaches at least 100% the odds of their BMI being 30 or above (of them being obese) are microscopically small. Without combining both measurements this meaningful and motivating conclusion cannot be reached. Thus by using both, you'll have a vastly more accurate and complete picture of the client's obesity level than you'd have if you used only BMI.

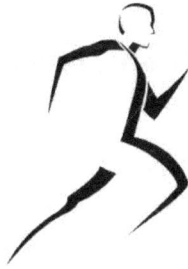

2

What Does a FORE Score Mean to Brad Pitt?

With three simple measurements you can generate a FORE Score for anyone including Brad Pitt. Here's how it works. With a tape measure attached to the wall, have Brad face the wall, reach up as high as he can, and record the point at which the tips of his fingers touch the tape measure. We'll call that the high measurement or POINT H.

Next with Brad facing the wall and the tape measure, record the point at which his chin touches the tape measure. We'll call that the low measurement or POINT L.

Now using a set of height adjustable pull ups straps, lower the grips to a point at which Brad can successfully complete at least one leg assisted pull up (jumping and pulling at the same time, stopping for a second at the top, and lowering himself down).

Leg Assisted Pull Ups

Presuming he can do several reps at this level, begin to raise the grips in small increments (you be the judge of small) and ask Brad to continue doing one more leg assisted pull up at each stop until you reach a point where he's unable to successfully complete one good rep. Then record the highest point at which Brad was successful. We'll call that the medium measurement or POINT M.

Subtract, Divide, and Conquer

With points H, L, and M in hand subtract L from H in order to get X. Then subtract L from M in order to get Y. Divide X into Y and you'll generate a percentage that we'll officially call Brad's FORE Score. In other words Brad's FORE Score will be something like 48% or 56% or 73%.

What Does a 70% FORE Score Mean to Brad?

Now, knowing that a FORE Score of 100% means Brad can successfully perform at least one conventional (non-leg assisted) pull up, and that the ability to perform at least one conventional pull up means the odds of being obese are about the same as winning the lottery, what does a FORE Score of 70% automatically mean to Brad?

In my own experience it means that with a little more time and a little more work, Brad will achieve a 100% FORE Score and he'll be able to perform at least one conventional pull up.

Furthermore, as long as he maintains the ability to perform at least one pull up, the odds of Brad ever being obese are miniscule. In other words, a FORE Score gives Brad *concrete information* upon which he can take *concrete action* in order to actively avoid America's # 1 health threat, obesity – for life.

What Does it Mean to Everyone Else?

In this process, some participants will have to change their eating and exercise habits in order to achieve a 100% FORE Score. Others won't have to change either.

But in the end, the odds of anyone (including Brad Pitt) who has a FORE Score of 100% being obese are about the same as winning the lottery. In other words, show me 100 people who can physically pull their own weight and odds are I'll show you 100 people who are not obese. It's about that simple.

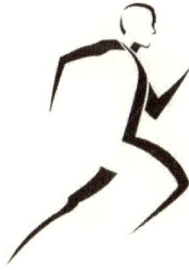

3

FORE Score's Big advantage Over Competitors

Aside from the omnipresent accuracy issues which we'll address shortly, the biggest downside to conventional body composition measurement tools (including hydrostatic weighing, the skin fold method, bio-electronic impedance, and of course BMI) is that they are all abstract and as such they offer very little in terms of motivational inspiration. Think about it. Have you ever seen anyone give a Tiger Pump over the opportunity to get their body comp or BMI tested? Odds are you've not.

The Big Downside of Conventional Measurement Tools

In all four cases they involve complicated formulas that are hardly ever understood by those who are being tested. Data is gathered, entered into the formula, which in turn generates a number that can be improved upon by eating better and exercising more.

But the frequency of change is so infrequent that almost no one is ever interested in retesting on any regular basis. And this lack of frequent feedback leads to a void in motivation and inspiration to keep on keepin' on.

Regular Return on Your Investment of Time and Effort

On the other hand, the FORE Score protocol revolves around a participant's ability to physically pull their own weight (do conventional or leg assisted pull ups). And when the stage is set correctly this strategy yields regular, tangible, documented, frequent feedback and improvement week after week for months on end.

The result of frequent improvement is that participants generate a consistent, predictable "return on their investment (ROI)" of time and effort. And as long as that investment keeps paying off, the motivation to continue investing remains strong. In fact it actually grows stronger (a phenomenon known in some circles as motivational momentum) instead of fading off into the sunset like the annual new-year's resolution.

Then There's the Issue of Accuracy

So the single most important advantage of the FORE Score tool over the competition is it's ability to motivate and inspire its users to eat better and exercise more until their respective goals have been reached. The second most important advantage is FORE Score's ability to yield accurate, meaningful feedback on body composition changes. That is to say when you lose fat or gain muscle, your FORE Score always improves. But when you gain fat or lose muscle, your FORE Score always deteriorates.

In contrast, BMI in particular is completely unable to distinguish between body fat and muscle mass. It throws all pounds into the general category of "weight" and it makes no attempt whatsoever to distinguish between body fat or muscle mass.

We confess that BMI has two major advantages over the conventional competition. First, it's significantly cheaper. And secondly it's universally accepted. And to be honest it's universally accepted BECAUSE it's cheap. The skin-fold method, electronic impedance, and hydrostatic weighing (in particular) are all so labor-intensive that they're too expensive to use in mass (i.e. in schools). Thus in this race, BMI wins by default.*

A Much Bigger Bang for Your Buck

Interestingly though, the labor-intensiveness and so the cost of generating a FORE Score is effectively the same as BMI. The big difference is that a FORE Score gives participants a motivational, inspirational leg up through frequent improvement. It also yields accurate feedback on body composition changes. And those are two huge advantages when it comes to winning the war on obesity!**

*There are also accuracy issues/problems with skin-fold, bio-electronic impedance, and hydrostatic weighing. Hydrostatic weighing however is the most expensive and is considered the gold standard by most exercise physiologists.

**At the original stages of FORE Score we suggest you use BMI + FORE in order to take full advantage of BMI's current universal acceptance and lack of expense. In the long run (when the public recognizes and understands FORE) we suggest that you drop BMI in favor of FORE Score exclusively.

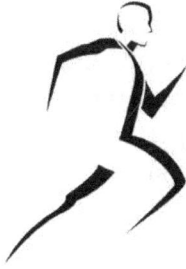

4

Vetting the FORE Score Concept

For what it's worth the FORE Score concept has yet to withstand the riggers of being officially vetted by a college, a university, a medical establishment, or a public health bureau. And we freely confess that we're looking forward to the day when that task is complete because it will allow a lot more folks to seriously consider FORE Score the preferable alternative to conventional options such as BMI or skin calipers.

A Logical Vetting

But in the meantime, and until the official, conventional vetting is complete, let's vet the FORE Score concept from a logical, practical, and an experiential perspective right now and see what we can come up with.

For starters, this concept revolves around a functional, body weight activity known as "Leg Assisted Pull Ups." The basic idea is to begin the learning process with LOTS OF LEG ASSISTANCE. Then gradually, over time, the leg assistance is reduced in small increments until it's no longer required. At this point the participant will have developed the ability to physically pull their own weight, i.e. to perform conventional pull ups.

Naturally Reflect Body Comp Changes

Now let's recognize that ALL body weight exercises (including running, jumping, skipping, hopping, climbing, and pull ups, etc.) naturally and automatically reflect changes in body composition through changes in functional performance.

For example, GAIN 20 lbs of body fat and what happens to your ability to run, jump, and do pull ups? It deteriorates, right?

Now lose that 20 lbs of body fat and what happens to your functional performance? It improves, automatically and naturally.

On the other hand gain 10 lbs of muscle mass and what happens to your functional performance? It automatically improves. Then lose 10 lbs of muscle mass and what happens to your functional performance. It automatically deteriorates.

This Doesn't Constitute News

None of these observations will constitute news to anyone. Exercise Physiologists would agree with them. Physical Therapists, Athletic Trainers, and the Strength Coaches would find nothing to argue with. Medical Doctors, Osteopaths, Chiropractors, and the Registered Nurses would shrug their shoulders and say "So what?" Junior high students would understand because they are so INTUITIVELY OBVIOUS.

But regardless of its obviousness, conventional minds demand an official blessing from conventional sources before they officially agree and recognize the truth in anything. And on one hand we applaud this conservative approach to medical matters.

On the Other Hand...

On the other hand, if you're sick and tired of pledging allegiance to concepts that have undermined kids from New York to LA, Miami to Seattle, you might be tempted to use the FORE Score concept in place of, or at least alongside BMI – because you see that, even without an official blessing, this concept gives you the accurate feedback you need to begin winning the war against childhood obesity in your school. If that sounds familiar, we say, by all means go for it.

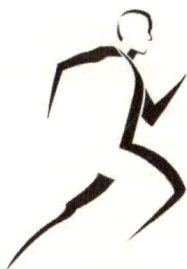

5

The American Society of Exercise Physiologists Endorses a Simple Solution to Childhood Obesity

Duluth, MN – Performance in exercises in which the participant's own body weight is the primary resistance (i.e. pull-ups, push ups, dips, and hand stand push ups) automatically improves when the participant loses enough body fat because the workload is reduced.

For example, a 150 lb. person who loses 25 lbs. would find it much easier to do pull-ups, jump higher, or run faster because they're carrying 16% less resistance. By the same token, the performance of a 150 lb. person who gains 25 lbs. of body fat will deteriorate because the workload has increased.

Exercises that use extrinsic, non-body weight resistance, (i.e. weights, plates, springs, and rubber bands) don't feature the same automatic performance feedback. Your bench press, for example, won't change just because you lost or gained 25 lbs. of fat.

Functional Acid Test Strategy (FATS)

This simple recognition has led to a new acronym in the field of childhood obesity prevention. Ironically it's called FATS which stands for *Functional Acid Test Strategy*. In the words of American Society of Exercise Physiologists President and former collegiate gymnast Dr. Tommy Boone, "Certain body weight exercises are challenging enough that obese people can't do them. Pull-ups, dips, and handstand push ups, for example, fall into that category."

One Example of FATS

So the FATS strategy suggests that a child choose one of those challenging body weight exercises as their own *functional acid*

215

test, and then learn to master it. One example is a program called *Operation Pull Your Own Weight* which says, "Kids who can do pull-ups are almost never obese. If you start them early, before they've had a chance to gain much weight, most kids can learn to do pull-ups in a predictable amount of time. And once they've learned to do pull-ups, they're immunized against obesity for life, as long as they maintain the ability." A simpler, more cost effective solution to childhood obesity would be hard to imagine.

Focusing on the Positive

The beauty of the FATS orientation is that it focuses on a child's strength development (all kids want to be strong at everything) instead of focusing on the negative and embarrassing concept of fat loss. With this extremely positive approach kids see it as cool, they buy in, and in a predictable period of time they can *naturally immunize themselves against obesity for life*.

Simple, Easily Documented, and Affordable

In Boone's words, "At ASEP we endorse active lifestyles and nutritious eating habits across the board. But we believe that the simplicity and positive character of the FATS orientation to childhood obesity prevention has something special to bring to this long and frustrating debate. It could be what we've been looking for all along. It's simple, easily implemented, documented, and affordable. Those kinds of assets are hard to beat these days."

www.ingramcontent.com/pod-product-compliance
Lightning Source LLC
Chambersburg PA
CBHW031156270326
41931CB00006B/295